The Essentials of Neuroanatomy

The Essentials of Neuroanatomy

The Essentials
of Neuroanatomy

G. A. G. Mitchell
O.B.E., T.D., Ch.M., D.Sc., F.R.C.S.

D. Mayor
M.B., Ch.B., B.Sc., F.R.C.S.E.

FOURTH EDITION

CHURCHILL LIVINGSTONE
EDINBURGH LONDON MELBOURNE AND NEW YORK 1983

CHURCHILL LIVINGSTONE
Medical Division of Longman Group Limited

Distributed in the United States of America by
Longman Inc., 1560 Broadway, New York, N.Y.
10036 and by associated companies, branches and
representatives throughout the world.

First edition 1966
Second edition 1971
Third edition 1977
Fourth edition 1983

ISBN 0443 02450 2

British Library Cataloguing in Publication Data
Mitchell, G.A.G.
    The essentials of neuroanatomy. — 4th ed.
    — (Churchill Livingstone medical text)
    1. Neuroanatomy
    I. Title   II. Mayor, D.
    611'.8   QM451

Library of Congress Cataloging in Publication Data
Mitchell, G.A.G.
    The essentials of neuroanatomy.
    (Churchill Livingstone medical text)
    Includes bibliographical references and index.
    1. Neuroanatomy. I. Mayor, D. II. Title.
III. Series. [DNLM: 1. Nervous system — Anatomy and
histology. WL 101 M681e]
QM451.M36   1983   611'.8   82-9688

Printed in Singapore by Huntsmen Offset Printing Pte Ltd

Preface to the Fourth Edition

In preparing the fourth edition of this account of the central nervous system modifications and improvements have been made to several figures and to the text without any significant alteration in the overall length of the work. The most obvious changes are in the terminology used which is based on the fourth edition of the *Nomina Anatomica*. However, in many instances the older and more familiar term has been retained in brackets for comparison.

We are grateful to Sue Jacobs and Peter G. Jack, Department of Teaching Media, University of Southampton, for help with the illustrations, to Mrs M.F. Pryce-Jones for typing the revised manuscript, and to the staff of Churchill Livingstone for advice in the preparation of this edition.

Manchester and Southampton, 1983   G.A.G.M.
                                                     D.M.

From Preface to the First Edition

This simple account of the central nervous system was first published privately (Morris & Yeaman, Manchester) 16 years ago for the use of my own students. It attracted a wider audience, however, and I received so many requests for copies that I decided to publish it more widely.

Our knowledge of the nervous system has increased enormously in the past 50 years and this is reflected in the ever-lengthening sections devoted to it in textbooks and by the appearance of specialized monographs. Most of these are excellent, but they are more suitable as works of reference and it is difficult for students to sift the essentials from the mass of information provided. One has attempted to make such a selection on their behalf and some of the more important facts about function and applied anatomy have been added: (the terminology used conforms to the international nomenclature, Nomina Anatomica, Editor G. A. G. Mitchell, Excerpta Medica Foundation, 1966).

It is a pleasure to record my thanks to Dr. E. R. A. Cooper, Dr. E. L. Patterson and Dr. G. T. Ashley for their advice on various matters; to Dr. J. H. Scott and Professor A. D. Dixon for permission to produce diagrams from their *Anatomy for Students of Dentistry* (Figs. 14, 19, 20, 21, 41, 44 and 55 in this edition), to Miss M. Gillison for Figs. 2, 3, 4, 5, 8 and 12 which are taken from her *A History of the Body Tissues* and to Professor Wilder Penfield for Figs. 31 and 34 from his *The Cerebral Cortex of Man*; to Mrs J. E. Kern and F. Kern for secretarial and other help; to Mr G. Wilson and the staff of the Medical Library; to Mr R. F. Neave who prepared some of the illustrations; to Mr C. K. Pearson and Mr P. Howarth for technical and photographic help; and to Messrs E. and S. Livingstone for placing so freely at my disposal their great experience in medical publication.

Manchester, 1966   G. A. G. Mitchell

Contents

Contents

The essentials of neuroanatomy

GENERAL ARRANGEMENT AND EVOLUTION

The nervous system consists of *central* and *peripheral* parts. The former comprises the brain and spinal cord, which are connected to structures in every part of the body by peripheral nerves containing *afferent* and *efferent* fibres. The afferent nerve fibres convey sensory impulses from the skin, muscles, bones, joints, vessels, viscera and special sense organs to different parts of the central nervous system where they are decoded and correlated. As a result, fresh impulses are initiated in the central nervous system which are transmitted by the efferent nerve fibres in peripheral nerves to the muscles, vessels and organs; these efferent impulses produce an appropriate response (based on the nature of the information resulting from afferent impulses) such as muscular contraction or relaxation, glandular secretion or inhibition, and increase or decrease in cardiac, respiratory, alimentary and other bodily activities. The possession of a nervous system therefore endows animals with the ability to appreciate and to react to their environment and provides the means to control the internal state of their bodies. This master system regulates and integrates the activities of all the other bodily systems for the benefit of the organism as a whole.

The simplest forms of animal life, such as the unicellular amoebae, have no nervous tissues and the reaction to any stimulus is merely the expression of the inherent *excitability* of protoplasm. Rising one step in the scale, the simplest multicellular organisms show early evidences of cellular specialization. Some cells develop contractile properties and the surface or ectodermal cells form a protective cuticle. A few of the latter become further specialized to appreciate changes in the environment of the organism and these primitive cuticular sensory cells send out delicate processes from their deep surfaces which make contacts with the contractile or motor cells (Fig. 1). These processes transmit or *conduct* the excited state to the contractile cells. Thus, the simplest form of *reflex arc* is

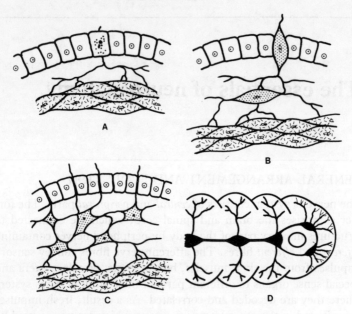

Fig. 1 Diagram showing evolution of simple types of nervous systems.
A. Primitive cuticuar sensory (receptor) cell forming contacts with underlying
contractile (motor) cells.
B. A receptor cell has sunk beneath the surface, but retains its contacts with
cuticular sensory cells and subjacent motor cells.
C. A more advanced stage of B in which there is a subcuticular ganglion cell
plexus.
D. Ganglionated chain seen in segmented forms such as worms, with an enlarged
'head' ganglion.

established, in which a sensory or *receptor* cell is linked to a contractile or *effector* cell and pleasant or unpleasant stimuli can now
evoke a suitable response, such as movement towards or away from
the source of stimulation.

A more advanced stage is reached when some of the receptor cells
sink beneath the cuticle, maintaining contact with the surface by
one process and making contacts with corresponding cells and with
effector cells by other processes. Such an arrangement is known as
a subcuticular ganglion cell plexus and it permits a local stimulus
to produce a generalized response (Fig. 1).

Rising still higher in the animal scale, segmented forms appear,
and the diffuse ganglion cell plexus becomes aggregated into a chain
of interlinked segmental ganglia which are connected by afferent and
efferent processes to the receptor and effector cells in their own segments. By this means stimuli applied to one segmental area may
provoke a co-ordinated response by all the segments and an element

of correlation of stimuli from external and internal sources is possible – a primitive form of integration. As segmented forms are elongated and move predominantly in one direction, the receptor apparatus at the advancing or head end receives a higher number of stimuli and the ganglion in the foremost segment becomes relatively enlarged to deal with these impulses. This ganglionic enlargement at the forward or head end is the first indication of the development of a supreme centre of control and may be regarded as the most lowly form of brain. Up to this level in the animal world the nervous system is still relatively simple, so that the responses to the same stimuli are almost instantaneous and stereotyped, while gradations of behaviour based on the lessons of previous experience are lacking.

The evolution of higher forms, and particularly of the vertebrates, required the elaboration of more and more complex nervous systems. The acquisition of special senses such as sight, smell, taste and hearing necessitated increases both in size and complexity, since these special sensory impressions had to be correlated with afferent impulses from the skin and deeper structures, and all had to be linked to their neighbours and to the effector side of the system by nerve pathways of ever-increasing complexity. The higher animals have acquired yet another characteristic – the ability to memorize experiences and to use them for future guidance. This has entailed great expansion of the so-called association areas of the brain, a highly important development most evident in the nervous system of Man. In consequence the possible reactions or responses of the higher animals to stimuli are almost infinite in their variety and gradations; their behaviour is no longer automatic and stereotyped as in lower forms, but purposive, controlled and protean. It is intelligent rather than instinctive.

NEUROGLIA AND NEURONS

The nervous tissues are composed of billions of nerve cells and their processes – *neurons* – supported in the brain and spinal cord by a special variety of connective tissue known as *neuroglia*.

Neuroglia
This is the supporting tissue of the brain and spinal cord and consists of three main types of cells:

1. *Astrocytes*
These have many radiating processes, some of which end on nerve cells and others on capillaries. They are neurectodermal in origin

and may assist in the transfer of nutrient and waste products between the neurons and the blood.

2. Oligodendrocytes

These are smaller and have fewer branching processes; they tend to lie in rows between nerve fibres. They are concerned with the production and nourishment of the myelin sheaths which surround axons in the central nervous system. Each oligodendrocyte is responsible for the myelin sheaths of several axons. These cells are neurectodermal in origin.

3. Microglia

These are diminutive cells which permeate the entire central nervous system. They are modified macrophages and form part of the reticulo-endothelial system and are probably mesodermal in origin.

Neurons

These are the *structural* units of the nervous system. They are mainly grouped in the brain and spinal cord, but other collections termed *ganglia* are found in association with various peripheral nerves. In mass, nerve cells are greyish in colour and areas of brain in which they predominate are referred to as the *grey matter*. Neurons are classified according to their size, shape, the type and number of their processes or on various other criteria. Thus they are described as small, medium or large (in man the range is between 10 and 200 μm); as spherical, fusiform, flask-shaped, pyramidal or multangular; or as unipolar, bipolar or multipolar depending on the type and number of their processes (Fig. 2). Neurons may also be classified according to their function, for example motor and sensory, or according to the chemical nature of the neurotransmitter which they utilise, for example cholinergic, noradrenergic or dopaminergic.

Each neuron possesses a nucleated cell body (the cyton or perikaryon) and one or usually more branching processes. The cytoplasm may be finely fibrillated and typically contains coarse or finely granular material which stains darkly with basic dyes, such as methylene blue, called Nissl substance. Many neurons also contain larger, more spherical, basophilic structures loosely referred to as dense bodies. In certain areas of the brain some neuronal cell bodies contain naturally occurring pigments such as melanin granules. The nucleus and its nucleolus (nucleoli) are well defined. The basophilic granular material or Nissl substance consists of endoplasmic reticulum with attached ribosomes (rough endoplasmic reticulum) and free ribosomes. It is found in the cell body of the neuron and dendrites but is absent from the region which gives rise to the axon, i.e. the axon hillock, and from the axon itself. Many of the dense bodies referred to above may be lysosomes. The cytoplasm of the neuronal

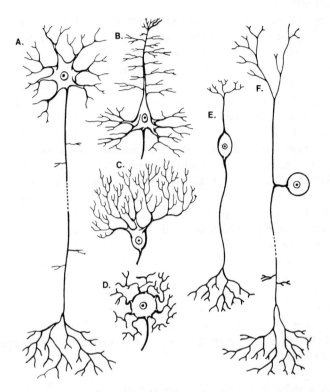

Fig. 2 Diagram of various types of neurons

A. Multipolar – these have multangular cell bodies with one axon and numerous dendrites. They constitute the majority of the nerve cells within the central nervous system.

B. Pyramidal – really a variety of multipolar neuron with a pyramidal shaped body. Typical examples are found in the cerebral cortex, and large ones exist in the precentral (motor) gyrus.

C. Flask-shaped cells – these cells are peculiar to the cerebellar cortex and their dendrites are notable for their rich arborescence.

D. Ganglion cell – the spherical type illustrated is commonly found in autonomic ganglia.

E. Bipolar – these neurons are afferent in type and have two processes. The one carrying impulses towards the cell is classed as a dendrite and the other, transmitting impulses away from the cell, is the axon. They are relatively uncommon types and are found mainly in association with special sense organs.

F. Unipolar (pseudo-unipolar) – In these the processes of embryonic bipolar cells have become approximated and apparently fused over a short distance and the single process soon bifurcates in a T-shaped fashion. They are afferent in function and are found, for example, in the ganglia on the dorsal roots of the spinal nerves.

cell body also contains numerous mitochondria, prominent Golgi complexes, a variety of tubular and vesicular profiles of smooth endoplasmic reticulum, microtubules and microfilaments (neurofilaments).

The neuronal processes are extensions of the cell body which conduct impulses to or from the cyton. They vary in length from a few microns to a metre or more; the longest interconnect the brain and the lower end of the spinal cord or extend to and from the cord in the nerves supplying peripheral structures such as hands and feet. One process conducts impulses away from the cell and is termed the *axon*. It does not branch freely except at its termination, although it gives off side branches or collaterals by which it establishes interconnections with other neurons. Most neurons have a variable number of *dendrites* which conduct impulses to the cyton. They are usually relatively short, branch freely and extend widely in the brain substance. They increase the surface area of the whole neuron and thus enhance the scope for its being influenced by other neurons. Dendrites contain similar organelles to those found in the cytoplasm of neuronal cell bodies. Axons contain microtubules, microfilaments, mitchondria, endoplasmic reticulum and vesicles related to neurotransmitter substances.

Neurons whose axons transmit impulses to muscles or glands are motor or secretomotor and those conveying impulses from receptor structures are sensory; the former are often referred to as efferent and the latter as afferent because of the direction of the impulses they transmit.

Myelin and neurolemmal (Schwann cell) sheaths

The axons in peripheral nerves are protected and insulated by Schwann cells and their associated basement membrane material with or without the formation of a *myelin sheath* (Figs. 3 and 4). Those axons which do not have a myelin sheath but are supported only by Schwann cells are called unmyelinated axons while those which in addition have a definite covering of myelin are referred to as myelinated axons. However, near their origins and terminations myelinated axons lose their myelin sheath and are covered only by a thin layer of Schwann cell cytoplasm and/or its associated basement membrane. Axons are devoid of any covering where they form synapses or neuromuscular junctions. With the exception of the peripheral processes of afferent neurons in sensory ganglia, which in many respects resemble axons, other dendrites are usually unmyelinated and covered only by satellite cells analogous to Schwann cells. Axonal processes together with their supporting neurolemmal

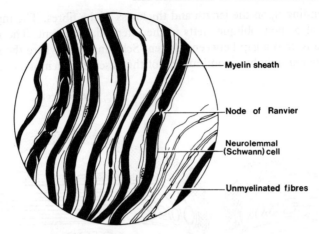

Fig. 3 Longitudinal section of myelinated (medullated) and unmyelinated (non-medullated) nerve fibres (× 210) treated with osmic acid which stains the myelin darkly. This obscures the enclosed axons, except at the nodes where the myelin sheaths are interrupted. Both types of fibres possess delicate nucleated neurolemmal sheaths.

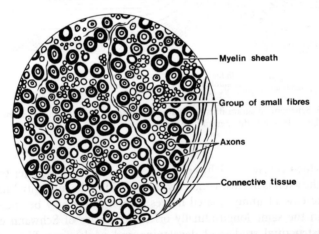

Fig. 4 Transverse section of a nerve (× 280) treated with osmic acid. The myelin (medullary) sheaths are stained black and the contained axons are white or pale grey in colour. The sheaths are very thin or apparently absent in the finest fibres.

(Schwann cell) sheath are often referred to as nerve fibres. In particular this term is applied to aggregations of axons which form tracts within the central nervous system and the collection of axons constituting peripheral nerves.

The myelin sheath is interrupted at the nodes of Ranvier (nodus neurofibrae) (Fig. 3 and 5) at intervals of between 0.1 to 1.5 mm depending upon the length and thickness of the fibres. The myelin may also show oblique clefts in the internodal segment. The node of Ranvier is a gap between adjacent Schwann cells where the axon is covered only by a continuation of the basement membrane mate-

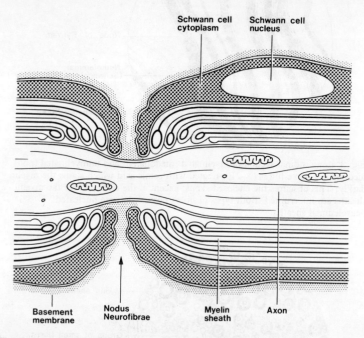

Fig. 5 Schematic diagram illustrating the arrangement of Schwann cell membranes on either side of a nodus neurofibrae (node of Ranvier).

rial which covers the Schwann cells. At the nodes of Ranvier therefore the axon is in close contact with the fluid in the interstitial space. In the case of unmyelinated nerves several axons may be enclosed within the same longitudinally orientated series of Schwann cells. Ultrastructural studies of developing and adult nerve fibres have shown that the myelin sheath and neurolemmal sheath are both derived from Schwann cells. The myelin is produced by proliferation of the plasma membrane of the Schwann cell which becomes wrapped around the axons. The thin layer of nucleated cytoplasm, together with the outer plasma membrane of the Schwann cell surrounding the myelin sheath, constitute the so-called neurolemmal sheath (Fig. 6).

In transverse sections unmyelinated nerve fibres are seen to consist of several axons invaginated into the cytoplasm of a single

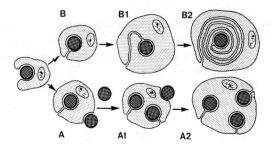

Fig. 6 Schematic representation of the relationships between neurolemmal (Schwann) cells and axons. A-A2 illustrate the invagination of several axons into the plasma membrane and cytoplasm of a neurolemmal cell to form unmyelinated axons. B-B2 illustrate the manner in which the neurolemmal cell spirals round a single axon to form a myelin sheath giving rise to a myelinated axon.

neurolemmal (Schwann) cell (Fig. 6).

In the central nervous system the internodal myelin sheaths are produced by the oligodendrocytes. Unlike the individual Schwann cells which produce the internodal myelin around a single axon, different processes from a single oligodendrocyte produce the internodal myelin around several axons. Consequently there is no cytoplasmic sheath surrounding the central myelinated axons comparable to the neurolemmal (Schwann cell) sheath in peripheral nerves.

Axons are more uniform in size than are their myelin sheaths. Unmyelinated nerve fibres consist of groups of small axons (0.2–1.5 μm in diameter) associated with a longitudinal chain of Schwann cells surrounded by basement membrane. The total diameter of myelinated fibres varies from 1 μm to 22 μm. The range in diameter of the larger fibres is mainly due to variations in thickness of their myelin sheaths. These differences in axonal calibre and overall diameter of myelinated nerve fibres are associated with different functional properties; for example, thin fibres conduct impulses more slowly than thick ones. Furthermore, these variations in fibre size and conduction velocities exist in both the peripheral and central nervous system. All axons are devoid of either cellular or myelin sheaths in the early stages of their development. Those axons constituting the tracts of white matter in the central nervous system acquire their myelin sheaths at different periods; indeed some do not become myelinated until after birth. Apparently the acquisition of a myelin sheath and functional activity are associated; for example, most nerve tracts concerned with visceral activities become myelinated before those which control the muscles responsible for voluntary movements.

Synapses

Within the nervous system impulses are conducted from one part to another along a chain of neurons. The terminal arborizations of the axon of one neuron usually ramify in close contact with the cell bodies or dendrites of many other neurons. They may also terminate in relationship to the commencement or termination of an axon. These structural and functional areas of contact, called synapses, may be axosomatic, axodendritic or axo-axonic synapses. The manifold contacts permit an extraordinary degree of integration and correlation. The special sites where axons 'synapse' with voluntary or striated muscles are called neuromuscular junctions or motor end plates. Although the relationships between neurons is close there is no true continuity between them in the central nervous system; the nerve impulse is conducted from one neuron to another by a chemical mediator or neurotransmitter substance which is released into the synaptic cleft between the presynaptic and postsynaptic membranes.

In general synapses consist of the slightly expanded ends of fine axonal branches called synaptic end bulbs or 'bouton terminaux'. When examined with the electron microscope the synaptic end bulb is seen to contain mitochondria, neurofilaments and characteristic synaptic vesicles which vary from 20–90 nm in diameter. The vesicles may be clear and appear empty or they may contain an electron dense core. Clear vesicles are believed to contain acetylcholine or some other neurotransmitter, while some of those with an electron dense core have been shown to contain a catecholamine. In some synapses the clear vesicles are rounded, in others flattened, a situation which may indicate functional differences between the synapses.

The concept that each neuron is structurally independent, although it has intimate structural and functional relationships with others, is referred to as the neuron theory. However, in the peripheral autonomic nervous system the proof that there is complete discontinuity at the termination of axons is not entirely satisfactory. The peripheral processes of neurons innervating viscera and vessels appear to unite directly to form a very delicate nervous syncytium, known as a terminal network or 'ground plexus'. The evidence that there is no real continuity between neurons is based on the findings that (1) some delay in transmission occurs at synapses, (2) normally the impulses travel in one direction only across these junctions as if the synapses acted as one-way valves and (3) degenerative changes in nerve fibres following injury to the cyton or its axon are confined as a rule to that neuron.

The fibres innervating the voluntary muscle of the body and limbs are the axons of large multipolar nerve cells located in the ventral horn of the grey matter of the spinal cord. It has been estimated that each of these motor neurons receives synaptic connections from the terminal axon ramifications of up to 1000 other nerve cells. All these synapses add their quota of influence to the motor neurons to the muscles, it is therefore appropriate that these large motor neurons and their axons are often referred to as *final common pathways*.

Reflex arcs
The *functional* unit of the nervous system is the *reflex arc*, a linkage of afferent and efferent neurons. The effector mechanism, e.g. a muscle, is supplied by an efferent nerve, and between the afferent and efferent components there may be one or more connector or intercalated neurons. These elements – afferent, intercalated (inter-nuncial) and efferent neurons – are the basis of reflex nervous activities (Fig. 7).

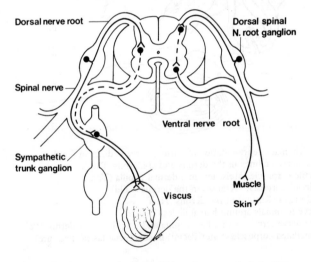

Fig. 7 Typical reflex arcs: somatic (right side) and autonomic (left side).

Some sensory endings are specialized and different types exist for the appreciation of different stimuli (Fig. 8). They are found not only in the covering layers of the body and in special sense organs such as the eye and ear, but also in deeper structures such as muscles and joints. The impulses engendered by stimulation of these endings are transmitted to the brain and spinal cord by afferent nerve fibres. Other sensory endings are simple, such as those for the appreciation

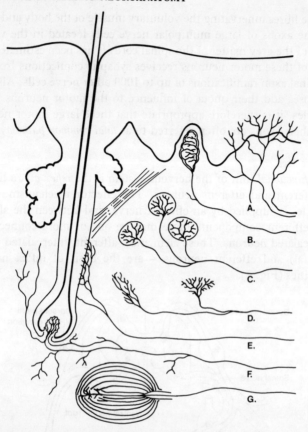

Fig. 8 Schematic representation of sensory nerve endings in the skin.
A. Free nerve endings in the dermis and epidermis (Pain).
B. Tactile corpuscle (Meissner) in a dermal papilla (Touch).
C. Bulbous corpuscle (Krause) in the dermis (Cold).
D. End organ (Ruffini) in the dermis (Heat).
E. Nerve terminals around hair follicles (Touch).
F. Free nerve terminals in a hair papilla and deep layers of dermis (Pain).
G. Lamellated corpuscle (Vater-Pacini) in superficial fascia (Pressure).

of pain in the skin and cornea, and consist merely of fine, free, terminal filaments of the afferent fibres.

Impulses produced from sources outside the body are termed exteroceptive (pain, touch, temperature, pressure, visual, auditory, olfactory and gustatory); those arising in the muscles, tendons, bones and joints are termed proprioceptive (sensations of movement and position); and those originating in the organs and vessels are termed interoceptive (visceral sensations of all types).

The efferent neurons convey impulses to muscles, glands and other active tissues, and in the simpler types of animals the reception of a sensory stimulus usually induces an immediate response in the associated efferent neurons, which in turn evokes an appropriate reaction in the effector mechanism. In higher forms the functioning of reflex arcs is less automatic, as they are controlled by brain centres which integrate impulses from both external and internal sources and sift them through the screen of experiences stored in the memory before initiating the appropriate efferent impulses. The presence of intercalated neurons permits both afferent and efferent components to establish functional continuity with many other neurons and an essential step in the evolution of the more elaborate types of nervous system was an increase in the number of intercalary neurons and linkages.

COMPONENTS OF THE NERVOUS SYSTEM

The nervous system is divided into *central* and *peripheral* components and these in turn are sub-divided into *somatic* and *autonomic* parts, but they do not differ fundamentally as they are closely interwoven anatomically and they consist of the same basic elements. The somatic part is mainly concerned with the reception of stimuli originating in the skin, muscles, bones, joints and special sense organs and with the transmission of stimuli to the voluntary muscles. The autonomic part is responsible for regulating the activities of the viscera and vessels and with maintaining constancy in the internal state of the body.

The *central nervous system* (C.N.S.) lies in the central axis of the body and comprises the brain and spinal cord. The former is composed of the cerebrum, the cerebellum, the mid-brain, the pons and the medulla oblongata. The spinal cord is relatively simple, but in the process of development the brain undergoes complicated changes (p. 115).

The *peripheral nervous system* consists of the cranial and spinal nerves which arise from the brain and cord, and of the ganglionated trunks, plexuses and nerves which constitute the peripheral parts of the autonomic component of the nervous system.

The brain lies within the skull and the spinal cord is lodged in the vertebral canal. The midbrain, pons and medulla oblongata are often referred to as the brain stem and connect the cerebrum above with the spinal cord below (Fig. 9).

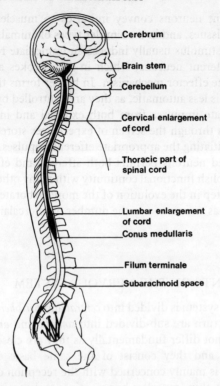

Cerebrum

Brain stem

Cerebellum

Cervical enlargement
of cord

Thoracic part of
spinal cord

Lumbar enlargement
of cord

Conus medullaris

Filum terminale

Subarachnoid space

Fig. 9 The brain and spinal cord *in situ*.

The spinal meninges

Both the brain and the spinal cord are enclosed and protected by
three membranes or meninges – the *dura mater*, the *arachnoid* and
the *pia mater* – which are directly continuous through the foramen
magnum. The dura or external coat is tough and fibrous, the arachnoid or intermediate layer is loose and tenuous, and the pia is a vascular layer of connective tissue closely investing both brain and cord.

The spinal dura mater is separated from the wall of the vertebral
canal by an *extradural space* containing fatty areolar tissue and a
plexus of veins. Between the dura and the arachnoid there is a
potential *subdural space*, but normally these two membranes are in
contact or separated by the merest film of a fluid resembling lymph.
Between the pia and arachnoid there is an important interval known
as the *subarachnoid space* which contains cerebrospinal fluid; this
space is directly continuous above with the corresponding space
around the brain and ends blindly below at the level of the second

sacral vertebra (Fig. 9). All three membranes invest the roots of the cranial and spinal nerves.

The cord is suspended within the dural and arachnoid sheaths by a regular series of triangular shaped projections from its pial coat which are termed the *denticulate ligaments*. These are attached in a continuous line on each side of the cord between the ventral and dorsal spinal nerve roots and extend outwards in the form of twenty-two pointed processes to become attached to the dura mater.

THE MEDULLA SPINALIS OR SPINAL CORD

The spinal cord on an average is 46 cm long and in the adult it extends from the foramen magnum to the level of the first lumbar intervertebral disc. Sometimes it ends about 2.5 cm higher or lower than this disc and it becomes slightly raised or lowered during flexion and extension movements of the spine. Above it is directly continuous with the medulla oblongata and below it ends in a tapering extremity, the *conus medullaris*. From the tip of the conus a slender thread, the *filum terminale*, is prolonged downwards as far as the coccyx. The cord is considerably smaller than the vertebral canal and this prevents any jarring contact between it and the surrounding bones. In general the shape is cylindrical, but the segments responsible for the nerve supply of the limbs are enlarged. The *upper (cervical) enlargement* corresponds to the fifth cervical to the first thoracic segments and the *lower (lumbar) enlargement* to the third lumbar to third sacral segments (Fig. 9). The segmentation is revealed by the attachments of the pairs of spinal nerves.

On cross-section the cord is seen to be slightly flattened antero-posteriorly, and it shows a central area of grey matter and a peripheral zone of white matter; the relative proportions of grey and white matter vary in different regions of the cord, the grey being more prominent in the cervical and lumbar enlargements which give rise to the nerves supplying the limbs. The cord is incompletely divided by a deep *ventral median fissure* and by a shallow *dorsal median sulcus* from which a *dorsal median septum* of neuroglia extends into the substance of the cord (Figs. 10 and 11).

The **grey matter** is mainly composed of nerve cells and their processes supported by neuroglia. When cut across it resembles an irregular H with *two ventral horns, two dorsal horns*, and a *central transverse bar* containing a minute *central canal*. In the intact spinal cord the grey matter forms a continuous fluted pillar and the parts appearing as horns on transverse section then appear as *ventral and dorsal grey*

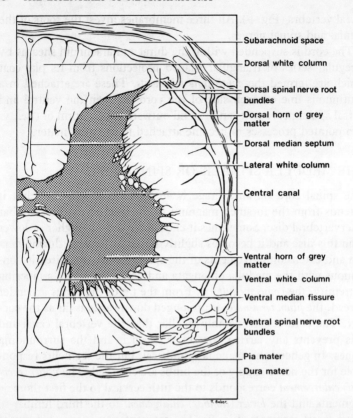

Subarachnoid space

Dorsal white column

Dorsal spinal nerve root bundles

Dorsal horn of grey matter

Dorsal median septum

Lateral white column

Central canal

Ventral horn of grey matter

Ventral white column

Ventral median fissure

Ventral spinal nerve root bundles

Pia mater

Dura mater

T. Baker.

Fig. 10 Transverse section through one half of the lumbar enlargement of spinal cord (× 13).

columns. In the thoracic and upper lumbar regions there is a lateral projection on each side, the so-called *lateral columns* of grey matter or *lateral horns* on cross-section (Fig. 11). The dorsal horn is capped by a crescent of semi-translucent nerve tissue termed the *substantia gelatinosa.*

The **white matter** surrounds the grey matter and is mainly composed of myelinated nerve fibres which are bound together by a neuroglial network. The white matter is demarcated into *ventral, lateral and dorsal (white) columns* on each side by the lines of emergence of the spinal nerve rootlets. The ventral white column lies between the ventral median fissure and the most lateral of the ventral nerve rootlets; the lateral between these rootlets and the dorsolateral sulcus marking the line of exit of the dorsal nerve rootlets; and the dorsal between the dorsolateral and dorsal median sulci. The two ventral

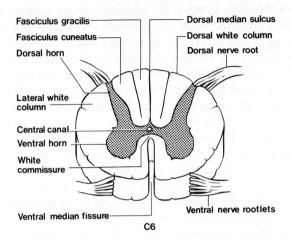

Fasciculus gracilis
Fasciculus cuneatus
Dorsal horn
Dorsal median sulcus
Dorsal white column
Dorsal nerve root
Lateral white column
Central canal
Ventral horn
White commissure
Ventral median fissure
Ventral nerve rootlets
C6

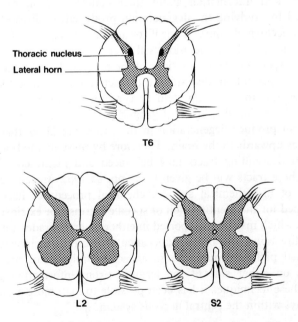

Thoracic nucleus
Lateral horn
T6

L2   S2

Fig. 11 Transverse sections of the spinal cord showing the characteristic appearances of the grey and white matter at different levels.

white columns are connected by a white commissure, which is the transverse band of white matter lying between the central grey bar and the ventral median fissure (Fig. 11).

Some of the nerve fibres in the white matter are confined to the cord, linking together its various segments and so they are termed *intersegmental*, while others are *commissural* and interconnect opposite sides of the cord. *Itinerant* or *projection fibres* connect the brain and cord, conveying impulses from one to the other and constituting various *tracts* whose fibres intermingle freely with those of the intersegmental and commissural fasciculi. Their course and identity have been determined mainly by two methods. Firstly it is known that the nerve fibres in different tracts acquire myelin sheaths at different periods and by appropriate staining of developing brains and cords the pathways may be charted. Secondly if the continuity between nerve fibres and their parent cells is interrupted in any way, characteristic degenerative changes occur both in the fibres distal to the point of interruption (Wallerian degeneration) and in the parent nerve cells (retrograde chromatolysis). Much experimental use has been made of this method in the identification of nerve tracts in animals, and information about their course in Man has been obtained by studying the degeneration produced by disease, operation or accidental injury. Thus if for any reason a group of cortical cells is destroyed degeneration will occur in their axons, and by studying specially stained sections of the brain and cord at different levels it is possible to determine the exact course of these fibres as they descend to the brain stem or cord. Similarly destruction of nerve cells in dorsal spinal root ganglia or of their associated nerve roots will produce degeneration in the ascending fibres that carry impulses upwards to the brain. Therefore by these methods ascending and descending tracts may be traced and identified. Details about these tracts will be given later (pp. 85–96). More recently a variety of histochemical and cytochemical procedures have been developed for the identification of specific intrinsic or extrinsic substances which may be transported in either an orthograde or a retrograde direction along axons. Experimental or traumatic interruption of axonal pathways may lead to an accummulation of such substances on either side of the lesions. From information gained using these techniques it has been possible to map more accurately pathways within the central nervous system.

Appearance of cross-sections of cord at different levels (Fig. 11)

Cervical
Cross-section large and oval in shape. Grey matter prominent,

especially in segments corresponding to cervical enlargement. The ventral horns in these segments are relatively large. The white matter is more plentiful than in any other region because the ascending tracts contain all the fibres collected at lower levels and the descending tracts still possess most of their fibres.

Thoracic
Section smaller and almost circular. Grey matter less prominent, but shows a lateral horn produced by an underlying intermediolateral column of cells. White matter intermediate in amount between cervical and lumbar regions.

Lumbar
Section again larger, due to an increase in the amount of grey matter in the segments corresponding to the lumbar enlargement. Lateral horn visible in upper one or two segments. White matter relatively less in amount than in the cervical and thoracic regions, because so far there are fewer ascending fibres and the descending tracts have lost many of their fibres.

Sacral
In the conus medullaris the grey matter forms two oval masses which almost fill the cord, there being only a small amount of white matter.

Location of cord in relation to vertebral spines
In early stages of development the cord is as long as the vertebral canal. Later, however, the vertebral column elongates more rapidly than the cord, so that by birth the cord ends at the level of the third lumbar vertebra and in the adult at the level of the disc between the first and second lumbar vertebrae. Thus, except in fetal life, the cord segments do not lie opposite the corresponding vertebrae but at varying distances above them, and it is usual to localize them in terms of the easily palpable parts of the vertebrae, the spinous processes. In the adult the following is a sufficiently accurate guide; in the cervical region the vertebral spines are one lower in number, in the upper thoracic region two lower in number and in the lower thoracic region three lower in number than the corresponding segments of the cord; e.g. the fourth thoracic spinous process is approximately at the level of the sixth thoracic cord segment. The lumbar, sacral and coccygeal segments are crowded together and roughly occupy the area between the levels of the tenth thoracic and first lumbar vertebrae.

The spinal nerves

There are 31 pairs (C.8, T.12, L.5, S.5 and Co.1) of symmetrically arranged spinal nerves. They are attached in linear series to each side of the spinal cord by ventral (anterior) and dorsal (posterior) rootlets; the former contain the efferent and the latter the afferent fibres. The rootlets coalesce to form the ventral and dorsal roots and these in turn unite within the intervertebral foramina to form the spinal nerves. Each dorsal root has a ganglion upon it close to its point of fusion with the ventral root (Fig. 12). These ganglia also lie in the intervertebral foramina, except in the case of the first and second cervical ganglia which lie respectively upon the neural arches of the atlas and axis, and the sacral and coccygeal ganglia which lie within the vertebral canal.

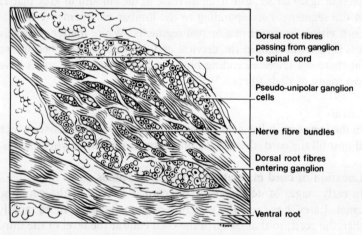

Dorsal root fibres passing from ganglion to spinal cord

Pseudo-unipolar ganglion cells

Nerve fibre bundles

Dorsal root fibres entering ganglion

Ventral root

Fig. 12 Section of a dorsal spinal nerve root ganglion (× 20).

Owing to the difference in the adult between the length of the vertebral canal and the contained cord, the nerve roots, which passed almost horizontally outwards in the embryo, retain this arrangement only in the upper cervical region. The others descend for increasing distances before they reach their appropriate inter-vertebral exit foramina. The lower lumbar, sacral and coccygeal nerve roots descend almost vertically in the form of a leash through the lower part of the vertebral canal and constitute the *cauda equina* surrounding the filum terminale (meningeum).

The spinal nerves formed by the fusion of the ventral and dorsal nerve roots are short. They divide almost immediately into ventral and dorsal rami which are responsible for the innervation of the skel-

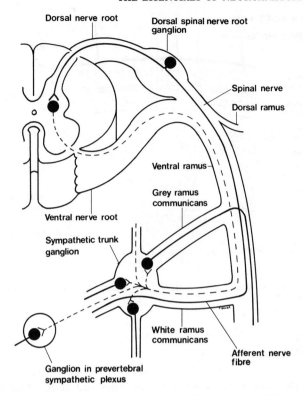

Fig. 13 Diagram showing the formation of a typical spinal nerve and its communications with a nearby sympathetic trunk ganglion.

etal muscles and the skin of the neck, trunk and limbs. Each ramus contains efferent and afferent fibres derived from the ventral and dorsal nerve roots, together with a variable proportion of fibres derived from the nearby sympathetic trunks (Fig. 13).

THE CEREBRAL MENINGES

The cerebral dura mater
The arrangement of the cerebral dura mater is more complicated than that of the cord, and its outer surface adheres to the inner surface of the skull and forms an endosteum. Therefore no extradural space exists between it and the skull comparable to that found between the spinal dura mater and the walls of the vertebral canal.

It consists of outer or *endosteal* and inner or *meningeal* layers, which are more or less closely united except along certain lines where

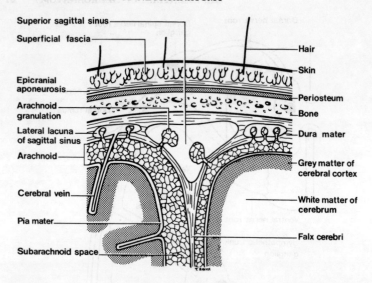

Fig. 14 A coronal section through the superior sagittal venous sinus and adjacent structures.

they separate to form endothelial lined channels, the *venous sinuses of the dura mater* (Fig. 14).

The outer surface adheres to the adjacent cranial bones, the adhesion being most definite along suture lines and at the base of the skull, and it sends numerous fine fibrous processes and blood vessels into them. Before the sutures close the endosteal layer is connected with the periosteum by the sutural membranes. These connections are obliterated as the sutures close, but the dura and the periosteum are still connected at the margins of the various foramina of the skull. The cranial nerves are surrounded by tubular sheaths of dura as they pass through the foramina of the skull and these fuse with the epineurium of each nerve outside the skull.

The inner surface of the meningeal layer is smooth and is separated from the arachnoid by the *subdural space*, a space in name only, since the dura and arachnoid are normally in direct contact. This layer sends inwards four strong septa which project into the cranial cavity and divide it into a series of compartments which communicate freely with one another and lodge subdivisions of the brain. These processes are: (1) the falx cerebri, (2) the tentorium cerebelli, (3) the falx cerebelli, and (4) the diaphragma sellae.

The **falx cerebri** is a sickle-shaped fold which lies in the longitudinal fissure between the cerebral hemispheres (Fig. 15). It is narrower in front at its attachment to the crista galli of the ethmoid

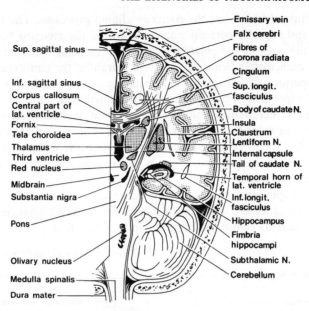

Fig. 15 Coronal section of half of the head passing vertically through the brain stem.

than behind where it is attached to the upper surface of the tentorium cerebelli. The anterior part is thin and frequently cribriform. Its upper convex margin lodges the superior sagittal sinus and is attached in the median plane to the inner surface of the cranial vault from the crista galli to the internal occipital protuberance. The anterior part of the lower margin is concave and free and contains the inferior sagittal sinus; the posterior part of this border is attached to the upper surface of the tentorium cerebelli and the straight sinus lies between them.

The **tentorium cerebelli** is a crescentic sheet of dura mater which roofs in most of the posterior cranial fossa and lies between the occipital lobes of the cerebrum and the cerebellum. It is arched upwards towards the falx cerebri, which is attached to its upper surface in the median plane. Its concave anterior border is free and forms an opening termed the *tentorial notch* which is occupied by the mid-brain. The anterior end of the free anterior border is attached to the anterior clinoid process. The posterior and lateral margins are convex and are attached to the lips of the transverse sulci on the occipital bone, to the postero-inferior (mastoid) angles of the parietals, and to the superior borders of the petrous parts of the temporal bones and the posterior clinoid processes. The transverse and superior petrosal sinuses lie within the attached border. Near the apex of the petrous part of the temporal bone the dura mater immediately below the attached margin of the tentorium and the superior petrosal sinus is evaginated to form a small recess, the *cavum trigeminale*, which lodges the trigeminal ganglion.

The **falx cerebelli** is a small crescentic fold of dura mater which projects forwards from the internal occipital crest into the posterior cerebellar notch. Its base is attached above to the under aspect of the tentorium and its apex extends to the posterior margin of the foramen magnum.

The **diaphragma sellae** is a small circular lamina of dura which forms a roof for the sella turcica and covers the hypophysis cerebri. A hole near its centre transmits the infundibulum (Fig. 16).

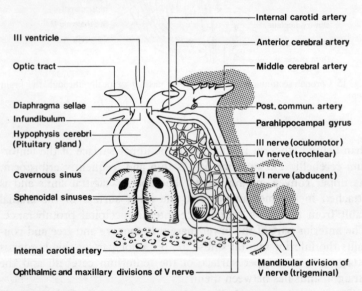

Fig. 16 Coronal section through the hypophysis cerebri (pituitary gland) and cavernous sinuses to show their important relationships.

The nerve and blood supplies
The dura receives its sensory nerve supply mainly from the trigeminal, vagus and first two cervical nerves through their recurrent meningeal branches; it is also supplied by sympathetic filaments which accompany the meningeal arteries and by parasympathetic fibres through the facial, greater petrosal and vagus nerves.

The arteries are derived from branches of the internal and external carotid and vertebral arteries. The *middle meningeal* branch of the maxillary artery (from the external carotid) is the largest of these vessels. It enters the middle cranial fossa through the foramen spinosum, passes forwards for a short distance in a groove on the greater wing of the sphenoid embedded in the outer layer of the dura mater, and then divides into anterior and posterior terminal branches. The anterior branch is larger and passes upwards to the anteroinferior angle of the parietal bone; *in this region it lies in a groove or tunnel in the bone and is liable to be torn in fractures of the skull vault.* It continues onwards towards the vertex, supplying branches to the adjoining bone and dura. The posterior branch passes backwards across the greater wing of the sphenoid and the squamous part of the temporal bone, giving off branches which supply the dura almost as far as the vertex and occiput. The middle meningeal arteries are closely accompanied by meningeal veins which lie between them and the bone.

The veins returning the blood from the dura mater anastomose with the diploic veins draining the diploë of the skull, and they end in the venous sinuses of the dura mater.

The venous sinuses

These are situated in certain situations between the two layers of the dura mater. They receive as tributaries the cerebral and meningeal veins, they form communications through *emissary* veins with veins external to the cranium and they drain directly or indirectly into the internal jugular veins. They have no valves, their walls are devoid of muscular tissue, and they are lined with endothelium. Some of the sinuses are unpaired (superior sagittal, inferior sagittal, straight, occipital and basilar) and others are paired (transverse, sigmoid, cavernous and superior and inferior petrosal).

The **superior sagittal sinus** (Fig. 14) lies in the attached, convex margin of the falx cerebri and runs from the crista galli to the internal occipital protuberance, grooving the adjacent parts of the frontal, parietal and occipital bones. Anteriorly it may communicate with veins of the frontal sinus or nose, or with the anterior facial vein. As it passes backwards the superior cerebral veins drain into it and it communicates with the veins of the scalp by emissary veins which pass through the parietal and other unnamed foramina. On each side it is connected with a series of irregular venous spaces, the lateral lacunae, which lie between the layers of dura mater. Arachnoid granulations project into these lucunae and cerebral, meningeal and diploic veins drain into them. Near the internal occipital protuberance the superior sagittal sinus usually deviates to the right side and is continued as the corresponding transverse sinus, the slightly dilated junction being known as the *confluence of the sinuses*; occasionally it deviates to the left and runs into the left transverse sinus.

The **inferior sagittal sinus** lies in the free, lower margin of the falx cerebri. It receives tributaries from the adjacent parts of the brain and meninges. It is continued as the **straight sinus** which occupies the line of junction of the falx cerebri and tentorium cerebelli; in front it receives the inferior sagittal sinus and the great cerebral vein, and, after receiving several other tributaries from adjacent parts of the brain, it usually ends in the left transverse sinus, but occasionally it may drain into the right transverse sinus.

The **occipital sinus** is a small channel in the attached margin of the falx cerebelli.

The **basilar sinus** consists of several intercommunicating venous channels in the dura overlying the dorsum sellae of the sphenoid and the basilar part of the occiput. It connects the inferior petrosal sinuses and drains through them into the internal jugular veins.

The **transverse and sigmoid sinuses** really constitute one channel, but different parts receive different names. Both transverse sinuses commence at the internal occipital protuberance and each passes outwards and forwards in the attached margin of the tentorium cerebelli to the mastoid angle of the homolateral parietal bone. They then leave the tentorium cerebelli and curve downwards as the **sigmoid sinuses** across the cerebral surface of the mastoid part of the temporal bone to the jugular foramen, where they end in the internal jugular veins. Both the transverse and the sigmoid sinuses groove the adjacent occipital, parietal and temporal bones, and *there is only a thin plate of bone separating the sigmoid sinus from the mastoid antrum and mastoid air cells*. These sinuses receive the superior sagittal, the straight and the occipital sinuses, besides other direct tributaries from the adjacent brain and meninges, and they communicate with the veins of the scalp and the back of neck through the *mastoid and condylar* emissary veins.

The **cavernous sinuses** lie on each side of the body of the sphenoid bone and they are crossed by so many fibrous bands that they have a spongy or cavernous appearance on section (Fig. 16). Each extends from the superior orbital fissure in front, where it receives the corresponding ophthalmic veins, to the apex of the petrous part of the temporal bone behind, where it divides into the superior and inferior petrosal sinuses. The internal carotid artery, surrounded by a plexus of sympathetic nerves, and the third, fourth, ophthalmic and maxillary divisions of the fifth, and the sixth cranial nerves are all embedded in the wall of the sinus.

The hypophysis cerebri or pituitary gland lies between them, the sphenoidal air sinuses are inferomedial, the optic chiasma is superomedial, and the anterior ends of the parahippocampal gyri are lateral. The two sinuses are connected by small intercavernous channels in the anterior and posterior borders of the diaphragma sellae and the cavernous and intercavernous sinuses are sometimes described together as the *circular sinus*. They receive the ophthalmic and inferior cerebral veins and the small sphenoparietal sinuses which run inwards along the lesser wings of the sphenoid bone. They communicate with each other via the intercavernous sinuses; with the supraorbital and anterior facial veins through the superior ophthalmic veins; with the pterygoid plexuses by emissary veins which pass through basal foramina (ovale, lacerum, etc.); with the transverse sinuses through the superior petrosal sinuses; and with the internal jugular veins via the inferior petrosal sinuses.

The **superior petrosal sinuses** are narrow channels lying in the attached margin of the tentorium cerebelli which connect the cavernous and transverse sinuses. Each lies in a groove on the superior border of the petrous part of the temporal bone.

The **inferior petrosal sinuses** drain the cavernous sinuses into the internal jugular veins and each descends in the groove between the petrous part of the temporal bone and the basilar part of the occipital bone. They receive tributaries from the inferior part of the cerebellum and from the internal ears.

The arachnoid

This is a delicate membrane which envelops both the brain and the cord, intervening between the dura mater and pia mater (Fig. 14). It is separated from the dura by the potential *subdural space* and from the pia by a definite interval, the *subarachnoid space*, which is filled with cerebrospinal fluid. It ensheathes the cranial and spinal nerves as far as their points of exit from the skull and vertebral canal.

The arachnoid mater is carried into the longitudinal fissure by the falx cerebri and into the stem of the lateral sulcus by the lesser wing of the sphenoid, but it bridges across the fissures and sulci; in places it is separated from the brain surface by wider intervals, the *subarachnoid cisterns*. The arachnoid and pia mater are connected by numerous fine strands of connective tissue which traverse the subarachnoid space. These strands are less abundant in the cisterns.

The *arachnoid granulations* are small excrescences from the arachnoid which project into the superior sagittal, transverse and some other sinuses, but mainly into the lateral lacunae connected with the superior sagittal sinus (Fig. 14). These granulations enlarge with age and cause pressure absorption of the overlying skull, so producing the small pits commonly seen in the vicinity of the groove for the superior sagittal sinus. Besides these macroscopic granulations there are numerous microscopic arachnoid projections into the dural venous sinuses. These are termed the *arachnoid villi* and the granulations may be regarded as greatly enlarged or aggregated villi.

The subarachnoid cisterns. The *cisterna cerebellomedullaris* or *cisterna magna* is the space formed by the arachnoid bridging over the interval between the medulla oblongata and the under surface of the cerebellum (Fig. 18). The *cisterna pontis* is a widening of the subarachnoid space in front of the pons and it is continuous with the subarachnoid space around the spinal cord below and with the cisterna cerebellomedullaris behind. Above the pons the arachnoid bridges across between the cerebral peduncles: this space is the *cisterna interpeduncularis* and the circulus arteriosus lies within it.

The subarachnoid space has no connection with the subdural space, but it communicates with the ventricles of the brain through the median and lateral apertures of the fourth ventricle (p. 46).

The **cerebrospinal fluid** is a clear, colourless, slightly alkaline fluid of low specific gravity. It is produced by the vascular choroid plexuses in the ventricles and passes into the subarachnoid space through the median and lateral apertures of the fourth ventricle. Some of the fluid passes downwards into the spinal subarachnoid space, but most of it flows upwards through the tentorial notch and ascends over the lateral surfaces of the cerebral hemispheres to be absorbed again into the bloodstream, through the arachnoid villi and granulations and through the walls of capillaries.

The pia mater

The pia mater (Fig. 14) is the very vascular membrane which closely invests the brain and cord, adapting itself accurately to their surfaces and becoming invaginated into the choroid fissure to form the tela choroidea (p. 76) of the third ventricle. The blood vessels on the surface of the brain lie in the subarachnoid space and many of their branches ramify in the pia mater before penetrating the brain substance. As they enter the brain they are invested by sheaths derived from the arachnoid and pia mater.

THE BRAIN

The brain is the expanded and highly complex upper part of the central nervous axis. It is enveloped by the meninges and is lodged within the cranial cavity, but whereas the vertebral canal is much wider than the spinal cord, the brain and skull are so closely apposed that the surface features of the brain impress themselves upon the inner surface of the skull. The average weight of the brain in a male adult is about 1380 grams (approx. 3 lb) and in the adult female it weighs slightly less. Male and female brains are proportionately equal, however, when related to the total body weight.

General appearance

When viewed from above the brain is ovoid, with the broader end backwards, and its widest region lies between the two parietal eminences. Owing to the enormous development of the cerebral hemispheres in Man, they alone are visible when the brain is looked at from this aspect.

The lower surface of the brain is termed the *base* (Fig. 17). It is uneven, being adapted more or less accurately to the irregularities of the base of the skull. Viewed from this aspect all the main divisions of the brain may be recognized – *cerebrum, cerebellum, midbrain, pons and medulla oblongata.*

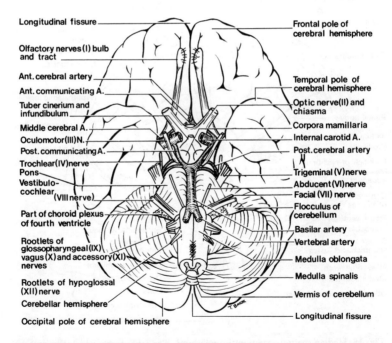

Longitudinal fissure

Olfactory nerves (I) bulb and tract

Ant. cerebral artery

Ant. communicating A.

Tuber cinerium and infundibulum

Middle cerebral A.

Oculomotor (III) N.

Post. communicating A.

Trochlear (IV) nerve

Pons

Vestibulo-cochlear (VIII nerve)

Part of choroid plexus of fourth ventricle

Rootlets of glossopharyngeal (IX) vagus (X) and accessory (XI) nerves

Rootlets of hypoglossal (XII) nerve

Cerebellar hemisphere

Occipital pole of cerebral hemisphere

Frontal pole of cerebral hemisphere

Temporal pole of cerebral hemisphere

Optic nerve (II) and chiasma

Corpora mamillaria

Internal carotid A.

Post. cerebral artery

Trigeminal (V) nerve

Abducent (VI) nerve

Facial (VII) nerve

Flocculus of cerebellum

Basilar artery

Vertebral artery

Medulla oblongata

Medulla spinalis

Vermis of cerebellum

Longitudinal fissure

Fig. 17 The base of the brain. From this aspect all parts of the brain are apparent but in Man, owing to the relatively enormous development of the cerebrum, it alone is seen when the brain is looked at from above.

The cerebrum

The cerebrum which forms the great mass of the brain is developed from the *forebrain* or *prosencephalon* (p. 119). It occupies the greater part of the cranial cavity, lying in the anterior and middle cranial fossae and extending backwards above the cerebellum, but separated from it by the tentorium cerebelli (Fig. 18). The bulk of the cerebrum is formed by the *cerebral hemispheres*, which are partly separated from each other by a deep median cleft, the *longitudinal fissure*. If the margins of this fissure are separated a massive bridge of white matter is visible in the depths, the *corpus callosum*, which is a great collection of fibres connecting the opposite cerebral hemispheres. The surfaces of the hemispheres show multiple convolutions (*gyri*) and furrows (*sulci*) arranged in an intricate pattern. The surface layers are composed of grey matter and constitute the *cerebral cortex*. Each hemisphere contains an irregular cavity in the interior called the *lateral ventricle*.

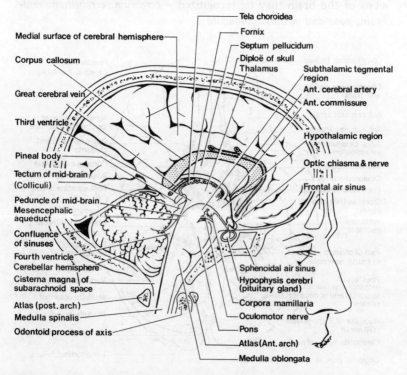

Fig. 18 Median sagittal secretion through head. The falx cerebri which lies in the mid-line has been removed to show the medial surface of the left cerebral hemisphere. The tentorium cerebelli is the double fold of dura mater interposed between the posterior part of the cerebrum and the cerebellum.

The inferior parts of the cerebral hemispheres are developed from the diencephalon (p. 120) which gives rise to the thalami (p. 69), hypothalamus (p. 74) and third ventricle (p. 75).

The cerebrum is connected with the parts of the brain in the posterior cranial fossa by the *midbrain* or mesencephalon (p. 38). This part retains more of its primitive characteristics than either the fore- or hind-brains. Anteriorly it forms a pair of *cerebral peduncles* connecting the cerebrum and pons. Its dorsal part is termed the *tectum* which supports four small eminences, the colliculi (corpora quadrigemina). Between them is a narrow tunnel, the *mesencephalic aqueduct*, between the third and fourth ventricles (Fig. 18).

The *pons*, the *medulla oblongata* and the *cerebellum* are derivatives of the *hindbrain* or rhombencephalon (p. 117). They occupy the posterior cranial fossa and are separated from the overlying cerebral hemispheres by the tentorium cerebelli. The pons is continuous above with the midbrain and below with the medulla oblongata which passes directly into the spinal cord at the level of the foramen magnum. The cavity of the hindbrain becomes expanded to form the somewhat pyramidal-shaped *fourth ventricle* (Fig. 18). It is convenient to commence the more detailed study of the brain by considering first the hindbrain derivatives.

The medulla oblongata

This is the direct upward continuation of the spinal cord and extends from the foramen magnum to the lower border of the pons. It lies almost vertically between the grooved surface of the basi-occiput in front and the cerebellum behind (Figs. 17 and 18).

It is just over 2.5 cm in length and at first is similar in girth to the spinal cord, but it expands as it passes upwards and so is shaped like a truncated cone. This enlargement is produced by the presence of new elements such as the olivary and other nuclei. The lower part contains a minute canal continuous below with the central canal of the cord, but this opens out above into the fourth ventricle.

The medulla oblongata is bilaterally symmetrical, a fact indicated by the presence of a ventral median fissure and a dorsal median sulcus.

The *ventral median fissure* is continuous with the corresponding groove on the spinal cord and it is interrupted at its lower part by bundles of fibres crossing obliquely from one side to the other – the *decussation of the pyramids*.

The *dorsal median sulcus* is continuous below with the corresponding sulcus of the cord and it is present only in the lower half of the medulla. Above its lips diverge to form the boundaries of a triangular area – the lower part of the floor of the fourth ventricle.

There are also *ventrolateral* and *dorsolateral sulci*, which are direct upward continuations of the corresponding sulci of the cord; along the former the rootlets of the hypoglossal nerve emerge and along the latter the rootlets of the glossopharyngeal, vagus and accessory nerves.

The sulci and nerve roots divide the surface of each half of the medulla oblongata into ventral, lateral and dorsal regions, an arrangement resembling that existing in the cord. But the constituents of the three regions do not correspond exactly with the corresponding white columns of the cord because a considerable rearrangement of nerve fibres and pathways occurs in the medulla oblongata.

The ventral (anterior) region. Between the ventral median fissures and the ventrolateral sulcus there is a rounded column known as the *pyramid*. It is most prominent above and the abducent nerve emerges in the groove between it and the pons. The lower end becomes less prominent and passes imperceptibly into the ventral white column of the cord, but only a small proportion of the pyramidal fibres actually enter this white column.

The two pyramids lie side by side, separated by the ventral median fissure, and they contain the motor fibres passing from the brain to the cord in the great *corticospinal tracts*. The majority of these fibres cross to the other side in the lower part of the medulla, thereby producing the *decussation of the pyramids*. The decussating fibres pass outwards and backwards and come to lie in the posterior part of the lateral white column of the cord where they form the *lateral corticospinal (pyramidal) tract*. The fibres in the lateral part of the pyramid remain uncrossed and continue downwards in the corresponding ventral white column as the *ventral corticospinal (pyramidal) tract* (p. 86).

The lateral region. Between the upper parts of the ventrolateral and dorsalateral sulci there is an oval eminence known as the *olive*, produced by an underlying nucleus of grey matter – the *olivary nucleus*. The lower part of this region is apparently directly continuous with the lateral white column of the cord, but in fact the continuity is incomplete, e.g. the majority of the corticospinal fibres are located in the lateral white columns of the cord but *not* in the lateral regions of the medulla, except below the level of the pyramidal decussation.

The dorsal (posterior) region. This lies behind the dorsolateral sulcus and, like the lateral region, it is divisible into upper and lower portions.

The lower part is continuous with the corresponding dorsal white column of the cord and contains the upper ends of the fasciculus gracilis and fasciculus cuneatus (p. 92). These fasciculi terminate at the level of the lower end of the fourth ventricle in the *nucleus gracilis* and *nucleus cuneatus*, which produce two small surface elevations – the *gracile and cuneate tubercles*.

Between the fasciculus cuneatus and the rootlets of the accessory nerve there is a third indistinct elevation overlying the spinal tract of the trigeminal nerve.

The upper part of the dorsal region forms the lower half of the floor of the fourth ventricle.

The internal structure of the medulla oblongata varies at different levels (Fig. 19).

In the lower part the appearance in transverse section resembles that of the spinal cord, but at higher levels additional nuclei appear and a rearrangement of fibres occurs. For example, about the mid level there are extensive motor and sensory decussations. The decussating fibres of the pyramidal (motor) tracts pass obliquely backwards and outwards through the bases of the ventral horns of grey matter and these separated portions of the ventral horns gradually diminish in size and disappear as they pass upwards, although a mixture of grey and white matter persists in the corresponding area which is termed the *formatio reticularis (reticular formation)*.

The substantiae gelatinosae capping the dorsal horns constitute parts of the *nuclei of the spinal tracts of the trigeminal nerves*. They are displaced laterally to a certain extent by the appearance of two additional horns of grey matter on each side which project dorsally into the dorsal white matter of the medulla. These become larger and more prominent as the transverse sections approach the level of the lower end of the fourth ventricle and form the *gracile and cuneate nuclei* in which the corresponding fasciculi terminate (p. 92). Fresh relays of fibres, the second link in this great afferent pathway, arise in the gracile and cuneate nuclei and constitute the so-called *internal arcuate fibres*. These fibres curve forwards around the central grey matter and then cross the midline, decussating *en route* with the corresponding fibres from the opposite side. Almost immediately after crossing they turn upwards and ascend as ribbon-like bundles, the *medial lemnisci*, which lie adjacent to one another, one on each side of the median plane, dorsal to the pyramids and ventral to the medial longitudinal bundles. This great sensory decussation occurs at a slightly higher level than the great motor decussation already described. As the lemnisci ascend through the brain stem their ventral fibres, and then the others in succession, gradually diverge from the midline, so that ultimately the ribbon-like bundles come to lie transversely with only their edges in contact.

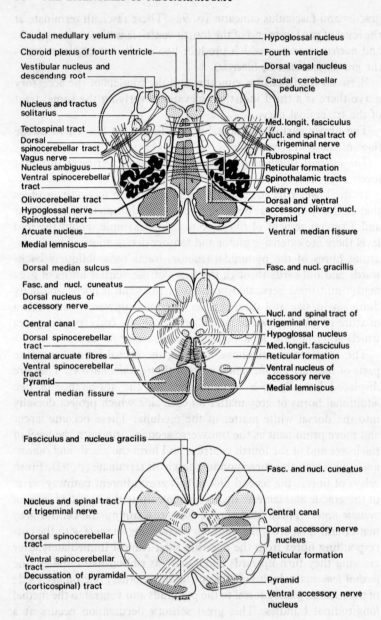

Fig. 19 Transverse sections through the medulla oblongata:
Top: at a level through the olivary nuclei.
Centre: at a slightly lower level through the sensory decussation.
Bottom: at the level of the decussation of the pyramidal tract.

Transverse sections through the upper half of the medulla show that the central canal has become expanded into the cavity of the fourth ventricle, the cuneate and gracile nuclei gradually fade out and other features appear, such as the various *nuclei of the eighth to the twelfth cranial* nerves inclusive, which all lie partly or completely in this part of the medulla, in addition to part of the *nucleus of the spinal tract of the fifth nerve*. But the most striking macroscopic features at this level are the *olivary nuclei*, which are convoluted laminae of grey matter underlying the surface projections of the olives and co-extensive with them. Each nucleus is bent in an irregular U-shaped fashion with the open end directed medially. Fibres (olivo-cerebellar) emerge from this open end and cross to the other side to enter the opposite caudal cerebellar peduncle. Additional smaller areas of grey matter, the *accessory olivary nuclei*, lie near the main nucleus and give rise to accessory olivocerebellar fibres.

The pyramids at this level form compact bundles on each side of the midline and their surfaces show a thin coating of grey matter, the *arcuate nuclei*.

On the dorsal aspect of the olivary nuclei and lateral to the lemnisci numerous tracts such as the ventral and lateral spinothalamic, the ventral and dorsal spinocerebellar, the spinotectal and tectospinal, the vestibulospinal, etc., are located (Fig. 19). These are described in the section on the nerve tracts (pp. 85–96). There are also two small but important tracts, the *medial longitudinal fasciculi* (Figs. 19, 20, 21). These lie close to the midline, dorsal to the medial lemnisci and ventral to the central grey matter. Each is a small bundle, continuous below with the corresponding anterior intersegmental tract of the cord, which can be traced upwards through the pons and midbrain in the same relative position to the central grey matter; a proportion of its fibres extend into the hypothalamus. These fasciculi may act as links between the cranial nerve nuclei, providing convenient pathways for the interchange of fibres between them and for the harmonizing of their functions. The essential co-ordination with the grey matter in the cord is effected through their continuity with the ventral intersegmental tracts.

The pons
The pons lies between the medulla oblongata below and the midbrain above, in front of the cerebellum, and behind the dorsum sellae of the sphenoid and the upper end of the basilar part of the occipital bone. It is shaped like a bridge (Latin, *pons*) (Figs. 17 and 18).

The ventral (anterior) surface. This bulges forwards and shows numerous small transverse ridges which indicate the disposition of the superficial fibres. On each side these transverse fibres become aggregated into a compact bundle, the *middle cerebellar peduncle,* which sinks into the corresponding cerebellar hemisphere. Above and below the pons is separated from the midbrain and medulla by transverse furrows.

In the midline anteriorly there is a shallow groove which lodges the basilar artery. This basilar sulcus, however, is not produced by the vessel, but by the downward passage through the pons of the two pyramidal tracts and the consequent heaping up of the overlying transverse fibres on each side of the midline. At the side of the pons and nearer its upper border the large trigeminal nerve emerges. An imaginary plane drawn downwards through this on each side marks the division between the pons and the middle cerebellar peduncle. The abducent nerve emerges through the furrow between the pons and the pyramid, and the rootlets of the facial and vestibulocochlear nerves appear between the pons and the olive.

The dorsal (posterior) surface. This is triangular in shape, forms the upper part of the floor of the fourth ventricle, and lies in front of the cerebellum. The lateral margins of the triangular area are formed by the two *cranial cerebellar peduncles.* Each emerges from its hom-olateral cerebellar hemisphere and ascends as a rounded elevation on the dorsal aspect of the pons. The two converge towards the upper end of the fourth ventricle and disappear under the caudal (inferior) colliculi. Their medial margins are connected by a delicate lamina of white matter known as the *cranial medullary velum.*

The internal structure of the pons (Fig. 20). On transverse section the pons is seen to consist of ventral and dorsal parts.

The ventral part contains both longitudinal and transverse fibres intermixed with small masses of grey matter, the *nuclei pontis (pontine nuclei).* It is best developed in the higher animals, an indication of the increasing importance of the cerebellum and of cerebral-pontine-cerebellar pathways as the animal scale is ascended.

The longitudinal fibres in the ventral part of the pons are the corticopontine and pyramidal tracts. The former are derived from cells in the frontal, parietal, temporal and occipital regions of the cerebral cortex and end by forming synapses with cells in the nuclei pontis. A fresh relay of ponticerebellar fibres then proceeds transversely through the pons and the middle cerebellar peduncle to the opposite side of the cerebellum. The pyramidal tracts contain corticospinal and corticonuclear fibres. These descend as bundles on each side of the midline, raising two rounded ridges which demarcate the basilar

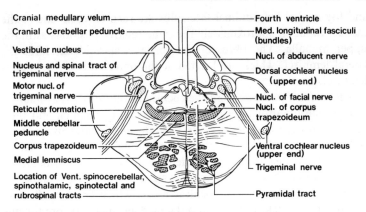

Cranial medullary velum — Fourth ventricle
Cranial Cerebellar peduncle — Med. longitudinal fasciculi (bundles)
Vestibular nucleus — Nucl. of abducent nerve
Nucleus and spinal tract of trigeminal nerve — Dorsal cochlear nucleus (upper end)
Motor nucl. of trigeminal nerve — Nucl. of facial nerve
Reticular formation — Nucl. of corpus trapezoideum
Middle cerebellar peduncle
Corpus trapezoideum — Ventral cochlear nucleus (upper end)
Medial lemniscus — Trigeminal nerve
Location of Vent. spinocerebellar, spinothalamic, spinotectal and rubrospinal tracts — Pyramidal tract

Fig. 20 Transverse section through the pons.

sulcus. They are less compact at this level than they are higher up in the midbrain or lower down in the medulla oblongata. Some of the pyramidal fibres (corticonuclear) do not travel as far as the cord; they decussate in the brain stem and form synapses in the motor nuclei of cranial nerves which send fibres to such voluntary muscles as those acting on the eyeballs, jaws, face, tongue and larynx. Other pyramidal fibres end in the formatio reticularis.

In the lower part of the pons there is a small group of transverse fibres, *the corpus trapezoideum*, which is distinct from the transverse fibres in the middle cerebellar peduncles. This group lies in the boundary zone between the ventral and dorsal parts of the pons and consists mainly of decussating fibres concerned with hearing. As they ascend the medial lemniscal fibres pass between and around the transverse fibres of the corpus trapezoideum.

The dorsal part of the pons contains most of the elements seen in the medulla. The central grey matter is spread out to form the floor of the upper part of the fourth ventricle, a number of new cranial nerve nuclei are present, the chief nerve tracts mentioned in connection with the medulla are all represented and the other areas constitute the reticular formation, consisting of islets of grey matter intimately intermixed with nerve fibres passing in various directions.

The cochlear, vestibular, abducent and facial nerve nuclei, the motor nucleus of the trigeminal nerve and the spinal tract of the trigeminal nerve and its associated nucleus are all found in this part of the pons. The facial nerve fibres form a loop round the abducent nerve nucleus in passing towards their point of superficial emergence between the pons and medulla.

The medial lemniscus, the spinothalamic and spinotectal tracts, and the medial longitudinal fasciculus are seen on each side of the median raphe in approximately the same relative positions as in the upper medulla. The fibres of the corpus trapezoideum form the lateral lemnisci, which are located at the outer ends of the medial lemnisci.

The *auditory pathway* from the cochlea to the cortex is as follows. The primary neurons are in the spiral cochlear ganglion and their central processes end in the ventral and dorsal cochlear nuclei in the pons. The secondary relay of fibres resulting from these synapses pass through the corpus trapezoideum and maybe also through the striae medullares ventriculi quarti (slender transverse bundles of fibres arising in the dorsal cochlear nuclei which cross the floor of the fourth ventricle and sink into the median sulcus) before turning upwards to form the *lateral lemniscus*. The fibres in the lateral lemniscus end mainly in the medial geniculate bodies, the *lower auditory centres*, and in the caudal colliculi. The new relays of fibres originating in the lower auditory centres pass through the homolateral internal capsule (p. 84) and auditory radiations to the auditory areas in the temporal cortex. Fibres arising in the caudal colliculi enter the tectospinal tracts and may be concerned with movements of the head in response to auditory stimuli. Some fibres from the lateral lemniscus end in the substantia nigra; others form synapses in nuclei associated with the lemniscus from which fibres enter the medial longitudinal bundle and so are conveyed to other cranial nerve nuclei. Certain fibres from the *vestibular* division of the eighth nerve and its nuclei may follow routes similar to the cochlear fibres and many vestibular fibres also enter the medial longitudinal bundle.

The midbrain

The midbrain or mesencephalon is the short upper part of the brain stem lying between the cerebrum above and pons below (Fig. 18). It is less than 2.5 cm long and consists of larger ventral and smaller dorsal parts; the former is formed by the two cerebral peduncles and the latter by the tectum. It is tunnelled lengthwise by an aqueduct which connects the third and fourth ventricles and lies nearer the dorsal aspect of the midbrain.

The tectum. The free surface shows four hemispherical elevations, the colliculi (corpora quadrigemina), separated by a cruciate depression. They are arranged in cranial and caudal pairs and they contain cores of grey matter. The pineal body rests in the groove between the cranial colliculi.

A rounded band or brachium is prolonged upwards and forwards from the outer side of each colliculus, so producing *cranial and cau-*

dal pairs of brachia. They interconnect the cranial and caudal colliculi to the lateral and medial geniculate bodies respectively. They are not prominent structures and are separated by a slight groove.

The cranial colliculi receive some fibres from the retina via the optic nerves and tracts and the cranial brachia, others which descend from the visual part of the occipital cortex, and still others which travel upwards from the cord via the spinotectal and spinothalamic tracts; the tectobulbar and tectospinal tracts originate in them and establish connections respectively with the cranial nerve nuclei in the brain stem and with the motor cells in the ventral grey columns (horns) of the cord in the cervical region.

Fibres reach the caudal colliculi from the lateral lemniscus and from the auditory part of the temporal cortex; some fibres originating in them pass in the caudal brachia to the thalami, while others descend to establish connections with cranial nerve nuclei and with motor neurons in the ventral grey columns (horns) of the cervical spinal cord.

The cranial colliculi are centres for one variety of visual reflex resulting in movements of the head and eyes in response to visual stimuli and the caudal contain centres for auditory and possibly vestibular reflexes in response to cochlear and vestibular stimuli.

The cerebral peduncles These are two thick rounded columns which emerge from the upper surface of the pons, diverge slightly as they pass upwards and forwards, and sink into the substance of the cerebral hemispheres. The medial surface of each peduncle bounds the posterior part of the interpeduncular fossa and is marked by an *oculomotor (median) sulcus* through which the corresponding nerve emerges. The lateral surface is related to the parahippocampal gyrus and shows a faint longitudinal *lateral sulcus*. The optic tracts wind backwards and the trochlear nerves pass forwards around the peduncles.

On section (Fig. 21) each peduncle is seen to consist of three parts: (1) a ventral part or *basis pedunculi*; (2) the *substantia nigra*; and (3) a dorsal part or *tegmentum*.

The *basis pedunculi* is semilunar in shape and is demarcated from the tegmentum by the substantia nigra. The two basal parts are separated from each other by an interval which is widest above. When each basis is traced upwards it is seen to pass lateral to the thalamus and to become continuous with the internal capsule (p. 84). Each is composed chiefly of corticonulear, corticospinal and corticopontine fibres; the two former constitute the pyramidal motor pathways already seen in the cord, medulla and pons and they occupy the middle three-fifths of the basis; the corticopontine fibres mainly arise

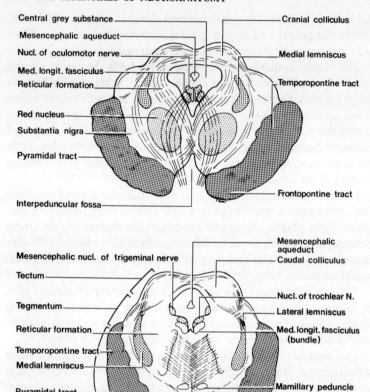

Fig. 21 Transverse sections through the midbrain:
Above and *below* at the levels of the cranial and caudal colliculi respectively.

in the frontal (frontopontine fibres) and temporal (temporopontine fibres) areas of the cerebral cortex and end by aborizing around cells in the nuclei pontis. From these nuclei new relays of fibres arise and pass to the opposite cerebellar hemisphere through the middle cerebellar peduncles.

The *substantia nigra* is a lamina of pigmented nerve cells lying in the boundary zone between each basis and the tegmentum. It is crescent-shaped, with its extremities reaching the medial and lateral sulci, and spiky processes project from its convex margin into the substance of the basis pedunculi.

The *tegmentum* is a bilateral structure and the division is indicated by a median raphe. Laterally the surfaces are free. Posteriorly the tegmentum blends with the tectum, except in the narrow line of the mesencephalic aqueduct.

The fibres in the tegmentum are predominantly ascending towards the cerebrum whereas in the basis the fibres are almost entirely descending. All the tracts seen in the dorsal part of the pons are represented in the tegmentum. The fibres of the cranial cerebellar peduncles decussate in the tegmentum before most end in the red nucleus, reticular formation and thalamus. The medial longitudinal fasciculus retains approximately the same position as in the pons, but the lemnisci are bunched together and tend to diverge from the midline as they pass upwards; the most lateral fibres (the lateral lemniscus) gradually incline backwards to reach the homolateral caudal colliculus and they may form a slight surface elevation, visible between the lateral sulcus and the caudal colliculus.

Surrounding the mesencephalic aqueduct, there is a thick layer of grey matter, the substantia grisea centralis, which contains the nuclei of the oculomotor (third) and trochlear (fourth) cranial nerves and the mesencephalic nucleus of the trigeminal (fifth) nerve.

There are two other important masses of grey matter in the tegmentum. These are the *red nuclei*, ovoid reddish masses which appear in the upper half of the tegmentum. Each is separated in front from the substantia nigra by a thin white lamina and extends upwards into the subthalamic tegmental region, while behind it is separated from the central grey matter by part of the reticular formation and the medial longitudinal fasciculus; laterally it is related to the medial lemniscus and the small ovoid subthalamic nucleus. Some of the fibres of the oculomotor nerve pass through it or lie in contact with its medial side.

Afferent fibres reach the red nuclei from the cerebellum via the cranial cerebellar peduncles, from the lentiform nucleus by striato-rubral fibres, and from various regions of the cerebral cortex. The nuclei give rise to rubrobulbar and rubrospinal tracts, which contain efferent fibres that end around cells in the cranial nerve nuclei and ventral grey columns in the upper half of the spinal cord; other efferent fibres end in the thalami and in the reticular formation of the pons and medulla. The red nuclei are important relay stations on the pathways between the cerebellum, the corpus striatum and the cord; these will be referred to again under the heading of extrapyramidal tracts (p. 88).

The reticular formation

Many tracts and nuclei in the brain stem and cord have been mentioned and illustrated, but considerable areas remain which show an admixture of criss-crossing fibres with larger or smaller groups of nerve cells (reticular nuclei) occupying the meshes – the *formatio reticularis*. Its ascending, descending and inter-connections are complex and incompletely understood.

Some collaterals from afferent fibres ascending in the spinothalamic tracts and lemnisci and others from the medial longitudinal fasciculi relay within the reticular nuclei. The axons of these reticular cells proceed upwards, and many or most of them form synapses in the small *intralaminar nuclei* located within the thalamic internal medullary lamina (p. 71). Projections from the intralaminar nuclei pass to other thalamic nuclei, to the hypothalamus, corpus striatum and cerebellum, and also to many or most parts of the cerebral cortex, probably via further relays in the *thalamic reticular nucleus* which is a thin layer of cells intermixed with the fibres of the thalamic external medullary lamina (p. 71). Various types of afferent stimuli can therefore activate this reticulo-thalamo-cortical system, producing a so-called arousal reaction unaccompanied by any definite conscious sensation.

Fibres from other reticular nuclear cells descend through the brain stem to the cord. Some relay in, or are interconnected with, other brain stem nuclei; others proceed further, often by a series of relays, and constitute reticulospinal pathways. A minority of the reticular nuclear cells have dichotomous axons, with one branch ascending to higher levels in the brain and the other descending to lower levels in the brain stem and cord. Some of the ascending and descending reticular connections described belong to the extrapyramidal system (p. 88) and so influence the activities of voluntary muscles, but others are concerned with autonomic and other activities.

Consciousness, attention, circadian rhythms and so on are not represented solely at cortical, thalamic or hypothalamic levels. Somehow they are dependent on correct functioning of the reticular formation. Any interference with it or its intricate interconnections following injury, disease or vascular disorders may produce alterations in the state of consciousness and/or motor, sensory and autonomic disturbances. Although the exact connections of the reticular formation have not yet been fully established, experimental and clinical evidence indicate their importance. Loss of cerebral cortical function for any reason reduces the person concerned to an automaton who is capable of a kind of vegetable existence. Somewhat similar results follow serious damage to the reticular formation, but in such individuals the vegetative state is usually transitory, for almost certainly they will also have sustained irreversible damage to 'vital centres', such as those controlling the cardiovascular and respiratory systems. Unlike the cerebral cortex, these 'vital centres' are essential for survival.

As stated above, stimulation of the reticular formation activates the cerebral cortex, altering its electrical responses and eliciting the arousal reaction. Localized stimulation of its component parts produces similar electro-encephalographic tracings to those associated with the conscious alert state. As nerve tracts conveying afferent impulses from body structures traverse the brain stem a proportion of their fibres or their collaterals end in reticular nuclei. Thus it is not surprising that stimulation of the reticular formation affects consciousness, since this state of attention and awareness is dependent on sensory information from many sources. Suppression of all afferent stimuli induces sleep.

The evidence therefore indicates that this reticular formation has many ascending and descending connections with higher and lower levels in the central nervous system and that it is involved in so-called reverberating nervous circuits between the brain stem, cord, cerebrum and cerebellum.

[*This section should be studied again after the various structures, systems, tracts, etc., not already mentioned have been described*].

The cerebellum

The cerebellum is the largest part of the hindbrain and occupies the greater part of the posterior cranial fossa (Figs. 17 and 18). It is separated from the posterior parts of the cerebral hemispheres by the tentorium cerebelli. It lies behind the pons and medulla oblongata and between them is the fourth ventricle.

It is ovoid in shape and consists of two *cerebellar hemispheres* united by a smaller median part termed the *vermis*. The distinction between the hemispheres is not very evident from above as in this area the superior part of the vermis forms a low median ridge. On the inferior aspect the two halves are separated by a hollow, the *vallecula*, and the inferior part of the vermis projects into this space (Fig. 22).

There is a wide ventral notch anteriorly which lodges the pons, medulla and fourth ventricle. The cerebellar peduncles enter the white matter of the cerebellum through the floor of this notch. Behind there is a narrow dorsal notch which lodges the falx cerebelli.

The surface of the cerebellum shows numerous parallel curved fissures separating narrow folia. The appearance is characteristic and quite different from the convoluted sulci and gyri of the cerebral cortex (p. 49). Only a few of these fissures need to be mentioned.

The *primary fissure* resembles a widely open V on the superior sur-

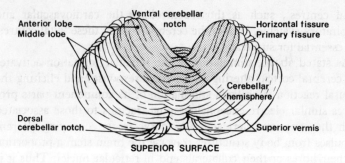

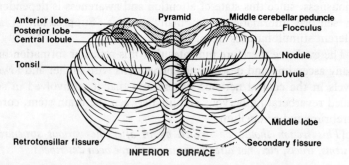

Fig. 22 The superior and inferior surfaces of the cerebellum. Various authorities have advocated complex cerebellar subdivisions, but here the older and adequate subdivision into three main lobes is retained.

face of the cerebellum, with the apex directed backwards. On each side the limbs cut into the horizontal fissure near the point of entry of the corresponding middle cerebellar peduncle; the primary fissure ends there and does not pass on to the inferior surface.

The *horizontal fissure* runs around the periphery of the cerebellar hemispheres, separating the superior and inferior surfaces; in front the cerebellar peduncles insinuate themselves between the lips of the fissure and push them apart.

The *secondary fissure* is a short transverse cleft which cuts across the inferior part of the vermis, separating the parts known as the *uvula* and *pyramid*.

The *retrotonsillar fissure* passes outwards from the vallecula opposite the secondary fissure and curves forward to end in the horizontal fissure near the flocculus. It helps to delimit a lobule on the inferior surface of the cerebellar hemisphere which is termed the *tonsil*. The two tonsils are connected to the single median uvula by a narrow strip of cortex, the *furrowed band*.

The flocculus
This is a small, ovoid, scalloped portion of the cerebellum which lies between the tonsil and the middle cerebellar peduncle. Each flocculus is connected medially to the *nodule*, the small portion of the inferior vermis in front of the uvula. Together they constitute the *flocculonodular or posterior lobe* which is phylogenetically the oldest part of the cerebellum; it is connected to the vestibular nuclei of the eighth nerve by vestibulocerebellar fibres.

Subdivisions of the cerebellum
Three lobes are described – anterior, middle and posterior (Fig. 22).

The *anterior lobe* occupies the anterosuperior part of the cerebellum above the entrance of the peduncles and in front of the fissura prima. It includes the greater part of the superior vermis, the anterior parts of the superior surfaces of both cerebellar hemispheres and the upper part of the ventral cerebellar notch.

The *middle lobe* is much the largest and comprises most of the rest of the cerebellum, i.e. the entire inferior surface and the greater part of the superior surface laying behind the fissura prima.

The *posterior lobe* is the flocculonodular lobe and is the smallest of the three.

The internal structure of the cerebellum
The cerebellum, like the cerebrum, consists of a central core of white matter surrounded by a grey cortex. This is the reverse of the arrangement in the pons and medulla, the other derivatives of the hindbrain. The peripheral disposition of the grey matter permits a vast increase in the number of nerve cells, an essential feature in the evolutionary expansion of both cerebrum and cerebellum. The nerve cells are chiefly found in the cortex, but there are also small masses embedded in the white central core. The cortex is broken up by numerous, curved fissures into narrow folia or ridges and these are further indented by multiple smaller grooves.

Of the deeper independent masses of grey matter, only one on each side, the *dentate nucleus*, is at all conspicuous. It consists of a convoluted U-shaped lamina located in the white centre not far from the midline. From the open end numerous fibres emerge and they constitute the bulk of the homolateral cranial cerebellar peduncle.

The white matter forms the central core and sends out numerous laminae and secondary laminae which project into the cortical grey folia. On section the branching appearance produced by this arrangement is characteristic and has been termed the *arbor vitae cerebelli*.

The fibres in the white matter connect different areas in the same cerebellar hemisphere or the same areas on opposite sides; that is, they may be association or commissural in type. They may also connect the cerebellum with other parts of the central nervous system and these projection fibres become aggregated together on each side into three bundles, the *cranial, middle and caudal cerebellar peduncles*, which all emerge or enter through the ventral cerebellar notch (pp. 94–96).

The fourth ventricle

The fourth ventricle lies behind the pons and upper half of the medulla oblongata and in front of the cerebellum (Fig. 18). Its tapering upper and lower ends become continuous respectively with the mesencephalic aqueduct and the central canal in the lower half of the medulla oblongata. On each side a narrow prolongation, the *lateral recess*, is carried outwards from its widest part and curves below the corresponding caudal cerebellar peduncle. The ventral end of the recess appears in the cerebellopontine angle, below the flocculus and behind the emerging rootlets of the glossopharyngeal and vagus nerves. The end of each recess is open and these openings form the *lateral apertures* of the fourth ventricle.

The fourth ventricle possesses lateral boundaries, a roof and a floor.

The lateral boundaries are formed on each side from above down by the cranial cerebellar peduncle, the caudal cerebellar peduncle and the cuneate and gracile tubercles.

The roof or dorsal wall is V-shaped as seen in sagittal section. It is formed above by the *cranial medullary velum*, a thin lamina of white matter filling in the interval between the cranial cerebellar peduncles, and below it is formed by the *caudal medullary velum*, an even thinner white lamina which stretches across between the caudal cerebellar peduncles. The lower part of the caudal velum is deficient so that a *median aperture* exists in the roof at this point. The median and lateral apertures of the fourth ventricle are the *only* openings through which the cerebrospinal fluid can escape into the subarachnoid space. If they are blocked for any reason the normal circulation of the cerebrospinal fluid is prevented and serious consequences such as hydrocephalus result.

The lower part of the roof is invaginated on each side close to the median plane by highly vascular tufts of pia mater, and the posterior walls of the lateral recesses are invaginated in a similar manner. These form the somewhat T-shaped *choroid plexuses* of the fourth

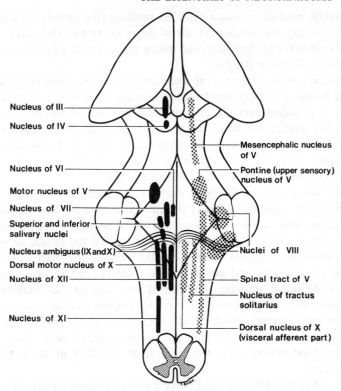

Nucleus of III

Nucleus of IV

Mesencephalic nucleus
of V

Nucleus of VI

Pontine (upper sensory)
nucleus of V

Motor nucleus of V

Nucleus of VII

Superior and inferior
salivary nuclei

Nucleus ambiguus (IX and X)

Nuclei of VIII

Dorsal motor nucleus of X

Nucleus of XII

Spinal tract of V

Nucleus of tractus
solitarius

Nucleus of XI

Dorsal nucleus of X
(visceral afferent part)

Fig. 23 Approximate locations of the cranial nerve nuclei in the brain stem. The motor nuclei are indicated in black on the left and the sensory nuclei are stippled on the right side.

ventricle, and small parts of the plexuses project through the median and lateral apertures.

The floor or ventral wall is diamond-shaped (Fig. 23) and covered by a layer of grey matter, which is continuous above and below respectively with the grey matter surrounding the mesencephalic aqueduct and the central canal in the lower part of the medulla. Its upper half is formed by the pons and the lower half by the medulla oblongata and it is divided into symmetrical halves by a *median sulcus*. The lateral boundaries are the cranial and caudal cerebellar peduncles.

On each side of the median sulcus there is a longitudinal elevation, the *eminentia medialis*, which is wider above than below. Immediately lateral to the upper part of the eminence there is a slight depression, the *cranial fovea*, and opposite the lower part of this fovea the eminentia medialis shows a rounded swelling (the *facial colliculus*) which overlies the nucleus of the *abducent* nerve and the fibres of the facial nerve encircling it: the motor nucleus of the *facial* nerve lies more deeply in the pons.

Several strands of fibres, the *medullary striae of the fourth ventricle*, wind round the caudal cerebellar peduncles, cross each half of the floor at its widest part and disappear into the median sulcus. They probably arise in the dorsal cochlear nucleus, reach the median sulcus as indicated, and then decussate in the pons with the corresponding fibres of the opposite side before joining the corpus trapezoideum and the lateral lemniscus (p. 38).

The lower part of the floor shows three triangular areas. The medial area is the lower end of the eminentia medialis and overlies the upper end of the *hypoglossal nucleus*. The upper part of the intermediate triangle is depressed and is termed the *caudal fovea*. The whole intermediate triangle overlies parts of the shared *dorsal nuclei of the vagus* and *glossopharyngeal nerves*, and is sometimes called the vagal triangle. The lateral area has its base directed upwards and subjacent to it lie the nuclei of the *vestibular* division of the eighth nerve, which extend both above and below the level of the medullary striae. Parts of the *trigeminal sensory nuclei* and the *nuclei of the solitary tracts* also lie deep to the floor of the fourth ventricle.

In addition to all the cranial nerve nuclei mentioned, 'vital centres' connected with cardiovascular, respiratory and metabolic functions are located in this region, besides multiple important tracts. It is not surprising, therefore, that even minor lesions in this small area may produce disastrous results.

THE FOREBRAIN

The relatively great expansion of the forebrain is a characteristic feature of the higher vertebrates and in Man the parts derived from it constitute the largest part of the brain. In primitive vertebrates sensations of smell are very important in influencing the response of the animal and thus the olfactory areas of the brain are prominent. In the higher vertebrates visual, auditory and all the other exteroceptive, proprioceptive and interoceptive impulses play an increasingly important part in determining functions and behaviour, and olfactory impressions become relatively less important. The enhanced value of the other varieties of sensation is evidenced by the expansion of the parts of the brain concerned with their reception and registration, and by the development of multiple new association pathways which connect these areas and permit integration of their activities. These cerebral elaborations reach their highest expression in the human brain and explain man's unsurpassed reasoning powers. This ability has placed him on a pinnacle in a world containing many more powerful animals, for brain always beats brawn.

The forebrain vesicle (p. 119) gives rise to the telencephalon and diencephalon (interbrain), and the former develops into the cerebral hemispheres.

The cerebral hemispheres
The cerebral hemispheres constitute by far the largest part of the brain and, when seen from above, they appear as an ovoid mass which is broader behind; the widest region corresponds to the part of the brain lying between the parietal eminences of the skull. The two hemispheres are partially separated by a deep median cleft, the *longitudinal fissure*, and are connected by a large commissure, the *corpus callosum*, which is visible in the depths of the central part of the longitudinal fissure. Each hemisphere contains an irregular cavity, the *lateral ventricle*.

The hemispheres are composed of an external layer of grey matter, the *cortex*, spread over an internal mass of mainly white matter. The cortex is the seat of the highest or intellectual functions of the brain, it is the level at which most of the sensory impressions received from the skin, body structures and special sense organs are consciously appreciated and it contains the areas which initiate and control voluntary movements. The cortex is not of uniform thickness, being thickest in the motor area and thinnest at the occipital pole. In order to increase the cortical area, the surfaces of the hemispheres show numerous convolutions or *gyri* and these are separated by fissures or *sulci* of varying depth. These begin to appear about the third to fourth month of intrauterine life. Before that time the surface of the developing human brain is as smooth as the brains of birds or reptiles.

The white centre consists of the myriads of nerve fibres which transmit impulses to and from the cortical nerve cells and from one cortical area to another. It encloses some larger and smaller masses of grey matter such as the *corpus striatum, claustrum* and *amygdaloid body* (pp. 78–80).

The surfaces of the cerebral hemispheres
Each hemisphere has three surfaces – superolateral, medial and inferior.
The **superolateral surface** is convex and conforms to the corresponding half of the cranial vault.

The **medial surface** is flat and vertical and is separated from its fellow by the longitudinal fissure and falx cerebri.

The **inferior surface** is irregular, being adapted to the floors of the anterior and middle cranial fossae, and behind them to the upper surface of the tentorium cerebelli. The front part is concave and rests on the roof of the orbit and to a lesser degree above the nose; it is termed the *orbital area*. The larger posterior or *tentorial area* is concavo-convex and lies partly in the middle cranial fossa and partly on the tentorium cerebelli, the fold of dura mater separating it from the cerebellum. The orbital and tentorial surfaces of each hemisphere are separated by a deep transverse cleft which is the stem of the lateral sulcus.

The three surfaces are separated by three borders – superior, inferior and medial, the last being subdivided into medial orbital and medial occipital parts. The superior border lies between the superolateral and medial surfaces; the inferior between the superolateral and inferior surfaces; the medial orbital between the medial and orbital surfaces and the medial occipital between the medial and tentorial surfaces.

The anterior rounded ends of the cerebral hemispheres are termed the *frontal poles* and the more pointed posterior ends are called the *occipital poles*. The prominent bulge at the anterior end of the tentorial area of the inferior surface, appearing below the stem of the lateral sulcus, is termed the *temporal pole*. About 3.5 cm in front of the occipital pole on the inferior border there is an indentation, the *pre-occipital notch* produced by a slight ridge on the upper surface of the tentorium cerebelli.

The convoluted pattern of the cortex varies considerably from brain to brain, yet there is a basic similarity in the arrangement of the gyri and sulci.

The **superolateral surface** (Fig. 24). Two important sulci on this surface may usually be distinguished without difficulty – the central and the lateral.

The *central sulcus* begins at the superior margin, a little behind the mid-point between the frontal and occipital poles, and runs obliquely downwards and forwards. It is sinuous and it ends above the middle of the posterior ramus of the lateral sulcus. Its upper end usually extends over the superior border to terminate in the paracentral lobule on the medial surface of the cerebral hemisphere. The *motor area of the cerebral cortex lies in front of the central sulcus and the somatic sensory area lies behind it*. The opposing walls of the central sulcus are themselves convoluted, the depressions and elevations on one side being adapted to corresponding elevations and depressions

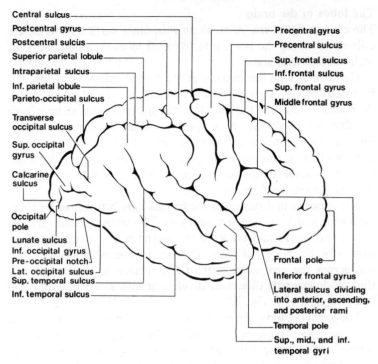

Fig. 24 Diagram of superolateral surface of cerebral hemisphere showing the main sulci and gyri.

on the other, and hence a number of subsidiary *interlocking gyri* are formed in the depths of the sulcus. This arrangement provides additional cortex without any increase in the lateral surface area and it is commonly found in other sulci.

The *lateral sulcus* is the most conspicuous of all the cerebral sulci and it appears on both the inferior and superolateral surfaces. It has a main stem and three rami. The part visible from below is the stem and it is a deep cleft intervening between the orbital area and the temporal pole; when the brain is *in situ* the lesser wing of the sphenoid bone projects into it. At its outer end the main stem divides into anterior, ascending and posterior rami. The *anterior ramus* is about 2.5 cm long and runs almost straight forwards while the *ascending ramus* runs almost vertically upwards for the same distance. The *posterior ramus* is about 7.6 cm long and extends backwards and upwards on the superolateral surface, to end in the inferior parietal lobule underlying the parietal eminence. When the rami of the lateral sulcus are opened up a buried island of cortex, the *insula*, is revealed (p. 52).

The lobes of the brain

The central and lateral sulci, along with other surface features, are utilized to divide the brain into so-called lobes – frontal, parietal, occipital and temporal.

The **frontal lobe** lies in front of the central sulcus and above the lateral sulcus. The **parietal lobe** lies behind the central sulcus, above the posterior ramus of the lateral sulcus, and in front of an imaginary line drawn between the pre-occipital notch and the parieto-occipital sulcus at the point where it cuts the superior margin. The **occipital lobe** lies behind this same imaginary line. The **temporal lobe** lies below the lateral sulcus and is bounded behind by the lower part of the above mentioned imaginary line.

The superolateral surface of the **frontal lobe** is traversed by three main sulci which divide it into four gyri. The *precentral sulcus* is often in two parts and runs parallel to the central sulcus, being separated from it by the *precentral gyrus*. The *superior and inferior frontal sulci* run across the remaining part of the surface in a forwards and slightly downwards direction, dividing it into *superior, middle and inferior frontal gyri* (Fig. 24).

The **parietal lobe** shows two main sulci and three main gyri. The *post central sulcus* is often subdivided and runs parallel to the central sulcus, being separated from it by the *postcentral gyrus*. The remaining and larger part of the lateral surface is divided into *superior and inferior parietal lobules* by the *intraparietal sulcus*, which runs backwards from about the mid-point of the postcentral sulcus; it usually extends into the occipital lobe and ends by joining the transverse occipital sulcus at right angles.

The outer surface of the **occipital lobe** is less extensive than the others and shows a few sulci. The *transverse occipital sulcus* is a short groove which lies almost vertically and forms a T-shaped arrangement with the end of the intraparietal sulcus. The *lunate sulcus* is short and curved, with its convexity directed forwards, and it lies in front of the occipital pole. The *lateral occipital sulcus* runs almost horizontally and the *calcarine sulcus* notches the occipital pole and appears for a short distance on the outer surface of the hemisphere.

The **temporal lobe** is divided by *superior and inferior temporal sulci* into *superior, middle and inferior temporal gyri*. The sulci run backwards and slightly upwards, in the same general direction as the posterior ramus of the lateral sulcus which lies above them.

The **insula** (lobus insularis) is a hidden portion of the cerebral cortex which has been infolded by the overgrowth of the adjoining cortical areas and it may be exposed by separating the lips of the rami of the lateral sulcus. It is triangular in shape and is surrounded by a groove which is named, rather inappropriately, the *circular sulcus*. The apex of the insula is antero-inferior and near the rostral (anterior) perforated substance. At this point the circular sulcus is indistinct or absent and the area is known as the *limen insulae*. The surface of the insula is divided into a larger anterior and a smaller posterior part by a *sulcus centralis insulae* which runs obliquely upwards and backwards from the apex. Each part is further subdivided by various shorter sulci. The claustrum and the lentiform nucleus lie deep to the insula.

The **medial surfaces** (Fig. 25) of the cerebral hemispheres are flat and they are mostly separated by the longitudinal fissure and falx cerebri, but they are connected in parts by cerebral commissures and by the structures bounding the third ventricle in the midline. They cannot be examined properly until these connecting structures are divided. When this has been done, the most conspicuous feature on the medial surface of each hemisphere is the cut surface of the *corpus callosum*, the largest of all the commissures, which appears as a flattened bridge of white fibres about 10 cm long, lying in the floor of the central parts of the longitudinal fissure. The main central part,

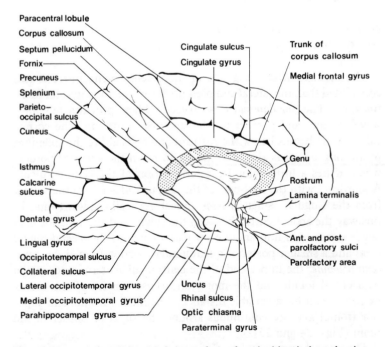

Paracentral lobule
Corpus callosum
Septum pellucidum
Fornix
Precuneus
Splenium
Parieto-occipital sulcus
Cuneus
Isthmus
Calcarine sulcus
Dentate gyrus
Lingual gyrus
Occipitotemporal sulcus
Collateral sulcus
Lateral occipitotemporal gyrus
Medial occipitotemporal gyrus
Parahippocampal gyrus

Cingulate sulcus
Cingulate gyrus

Uncus
Rhinal sulcus
Optic chiasma
Paraterminal gyrus

Trunk of corpus callosum
Medial frontal gyrus
Genu
Rostrum
Lamina terminalis
Ant. and post. parolfactory sulci
Parolfactory area

Fig. 25 Diagram of medial and inferior surfaces of cerebral hemisphere showing the main sulci and gyri.

the *trunk*, is slightly convex upwards. The anterior end is recurved downwards and backwards and is termed the *genu*. This tapers rapidly to form the *rostrum* which joins the upper end of the *lamina terminalis*. The hinder part of the trunk ends in an expanded, rounded margin known as the *splenium*.

Its superior surface is covered by a thin layer of grey matter, the *indusium griseum*, in which two delicate white strands are imbedded on each side of the midline, the *medial and lateral longitudinal striae*. The trunk is about one inch wide between the points where it sinks into the opposing hemispheres and the fibres spread outwards to all parts of the cerebral cortex of each hemisphere. The fibres of the genu curve forwards to the frontal poles and those of the splenium curve backwards to the occipital poles and on section they present U-shaped arrangements which are termed respectively the *frontal (minor) forceps* and the *occipital (major) forceps*.

In the midline posteriorly the trunk and splenium are attached to the body of the fornix (Fig. 25) and possibly to its commissure (p. 67). Further forwards the fornix diverges from the corpus callosum, leaving a triangular-shaped interval which is filled in by the *septum pellucidum*. The septum lies in the median plane and consists of two delicate laminae separated by a narrow cleft which has no connection with the ventricles. Its margins are attached to the trunk, genu and rostum of the corpus callosum and to the fornix (p. 67).

The medial surface (Fig. 25) of the cerebral hemisphere is less convoluted than the lateral and presents fewer sulci and gyri for identification. The *cingulate sulcus* is curved and lies approximately midway between, and parallel to, the superior border and the corpus callosum. It begins below the rostrum and ends above the splenium by turning upwards almost vertically to reach the superior border, where it lies a little behind the termination of the central sulcus. About level with the mid part of the corpus callosum another offset from the cingulate sulcus passes almost vertically upwards and in this way the area of cortex between the sulcus and the superior border is subdivided into an anterior part known as the *medial frontal gyrus* and a smaller posterior quadrangular portion termed the *paracentral lobule*; the upper end of the central sulcus terminates in the paracentral lobule and the motor and sensory areas of the cortex extend over it for a variable distance. The medial frontal and superior frontal gyri are continuous around the superior border of the brain (Figs. 24 and 25).

The curved gyrus between the *cingulate sulcus* and the corpus callosum is termed the *cingulate gyrus*; it is separated from the corpus callosum by the *callosal sulcus* and is continued behind the splenium as an isthmus on to the inferior surface to become continuous with the parahippocampal gyrus. At its anterior end this gyrus is separated by a slight groove from the small *parolfactory area*, which occupies most of the cortex between it and the lamina terminalis.

The posterior part of the medial surface shows two deep sulci which diverge from a point directly behind the splenium. The upper or *parieto-occipital sulcus* passes backwards and upwards to cut the superior border about 5 cm in front of the occipital pole, and it then appears on the surface of the parietal lobe for a short distance. The lower or *calcarine sulcus* corresponds fairly closely with the medial border of the hemisphere. It terminates anteriorly beneath the splenium, and the narrow area of cortex between is termed the isthmus and connects the cingulate and parahippocampal gyri. Its posterior end usually notches the occipital pole. The wedge-shaped region between the parieto-occipital and calcarine sulci is termed the cuneus and the area between it and the paracentral lobule is called the precuneus.

The **inferior surface** (Fig. 25) of the cerebral hemisphere is divided by the stem of the lateral fissure into a smaller, anterior, *orbital* part and a larger, posterior, *tentorial area*.

The *orbital surface* (Fig. 26) is slightly concave and rests on the roofs of the orbit and nose. It is marked by an H-shaped *orbital sulcus* and by a straight anteroposterior groove near the medial margin which lodges the olfactory bulb and tract and is therefore named the *olfac-*

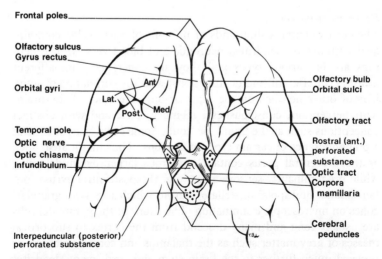

Fig. 26 The anterior part of the base of the cerebrum showing the main sulci and gyri on its orbital surfaces.

tory sulcus. The orbital sulcus demarcates anterior, posterior, medial and lateral *orbital gyri*, and the small convolution medial to the olfactory sulcus is the *gyrus rectus.*

The *tentorial surface* lies partly on the floor of the middle cranial fossa and partly on the *tentorium cerebelli.* It shows two anteroposterior grooves, the collateral and occipitotemporal sulci, which divide the surface into three more or less longitudinal gyri (Fig. 25). The *collateral sulcus* runs almost directly forwards from near the occipital pole, and anteriorly it may become continuous with the short *rhinal sulcus* which continues its line towards the temporal pole; in other cases these two sulci are separated by a narrow interval. The *occipitotemporal sulcus* lies lateral and parallel to the collateral sulcus and it is often divided into two or more parts.

The convolution lying medial to the collateral sulcus is termed the *parahippocampal gyrus* in front and the *lingual gyrus* posteriorly. The former is separated from a narrow strip of cortex, *the dentate gyrus*, by the shallow hippocampal sulcus, and the anterior end of the parahippocampal gyrus becomes recurved to form the *uncus* which contains the higher centres for smell.

The *medial occipitotemporal gyrus* is fusiform in shape and lies between the collateral sulcus medially and the occipitotemporal sulcus laterally.

The *lateral occipitotemporal gyrus* lies lateral to the occipitotemporal sulcus and is continuous with the inferior temporal gyrus around the inferior margin of the hemisphere.

Divisions of the cortex
The cortex contains thousands of millions of nerve cells, commingled with axons, dendrites, neuroglia and blood vessels. The neurons are of various types and they are concerned with afferent (sensory) or efferent (motor) functions; with the correlation of activities of other neurons on the same or opposite sides of the brain; with perception, consciousness, memory, etc.; and with abstract conceptions such as the 'mind' or 'soul'. Some cortical areas contain a preponderance of certain types of neurons. Thus motor areas such as the precentral gyrus contain numerous larger pyramidal cells, while predominantly sensory areas (e.g. the postcentral gyrus) contain smaller multipolar or stellate neurons which appear as 'granular' zones on microscopic examination. The axons of the pyramidal cells are usually long and many descend from the cortex to subcortical masses of grey matter such as the thalamus and corpus striatum, or proceed much further to the brain stem and cord; many dendrites from these cells pass horizontally, but a longer dendrite from each

pyramidal neuron often ends in the overlying layer of the cortex. The axons and dendrites of the smaller stellate neurons usually end within the cortex by forming synapses with pyramidal cells in adjacent layers.

The phylogenetically older areas of the cortex, such as those covering the piriform area and hippocampus (p. 67), are less complicated than the newer areas which include most of the human cerebral cortex. In the former, three layers can be distinguished – a superficial molecular layer of fibres with a few nerve cells, an intermediate layer of granular cells and a deep layer of pyramidal cells. The latter contain six strata (Fig. 27):

I.   The outermost *plexiform or molecular* layer consisting mostly of the apical dendrites of pyramidal cells and some intercalary neurons.

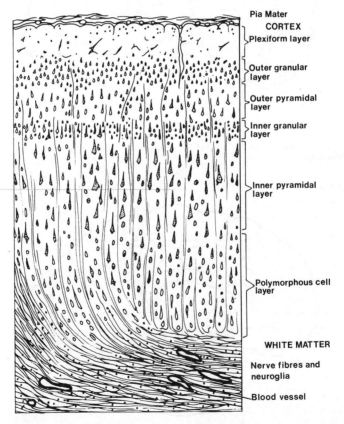

Pia Mater
CORTEX
Plexiform layer
Outer granular layer
Outer pyramidal layer
Inner granular layer
Inner pyramidal layer
Polymorphous cell layer
WHITE MATTER
Nerve fibres and neuroglia
Blood vessel

Fig. 27 Section through the cerebral cortex and the subjacent white matter (x 65) showing the various layers.

II and IV. The second and fourth layers are known respectively as the *outer and inner granular layers* because they each contain numerous stellate cells.

III and V. These layers are referred to as the *outer and inner pyramidal layers* because of their large content of pyramidal cells.

VI. The innermost or *polymorphic layer* is so-called because its cells are of many different shapes.

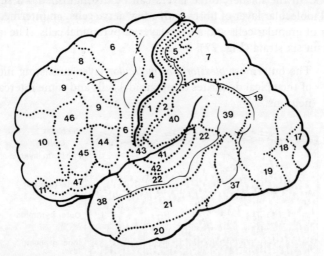

Fig. 28 Brodmann's cortical map of the superolateral surface of the cerebral hemisphere.

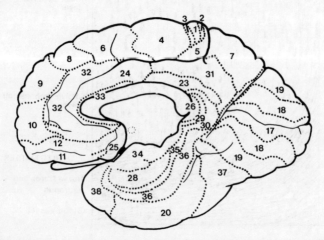

Fig. 29 Brodmann's cortical map of the medial and inferior surfaces of the cerebral hemisphere.

The areas of cortex covering the frontal, parietal, occipital and temporal lobes of the cerebrum are divided by sulci into gyri and these have been described. On the basis of detailed histological studies of the cells and fibres, the cortex has also been divided into multiple numbered areas which are represented on outline diagrams (cortical charts or maps) of the cerebrum (Figs. 28 and 29). These numbered areas do not correspond exactly with the gyri, and attempts have been made to correlate them with definite functions, but these have not been completely successful, for it is now realized that no cortical area is concerned exclusively with only one function. Nevertheless some gyri and cortical areas are concerned predominantly with certain activities and the information available will be reviewed briefly.

The frontal lobes
Information about their connections has accumulated as a result of operations on them for the relief of certain types of mental disorders and intractable pain.

The central sulcus between the frontal and parietal lobes is a *limiting sulcus*, separating the motor and somatic sensory areas of the cortex, the change occurring almost abruptly at the bottom of the sulcus. The anterior wall of the sulcus shows well-marked pyramidal layers containing giant pyramidal cells and poorly developed granular layers, whereas the posterior wall has conspicuous granular laters and less well-marked pyramidal layers.

The precentral gyrus constitutes the *motor area of the cortex* (Fig. 30) containing higher centres controlling voluntary or volitional movements of the *opposite* side of the body; the pyramidal (corticonuclear and corticospinal) tracts largely arise in them. The representation is *inverted*, with the areas for the head and neck inferior, and those for the leg and foot superior. The areas of cortical representation for the face and hands, with their finely graded movements, are relatively large (Fig. 31).

The *area (Broca's)* of the left inferior frontal gyrus around the anterior and ascending rami of the lateral sulcus controls the muscles concerned with speech production and is called the *motor speech area*. Lesions in this region produce motor aphasia (inability to control the muscles concerned in speech production). In left-handed persons this area is located in the right inferior frontal gyrus.

A proportion of the fibres arising in the frontal cortex belong to the *extra-pyramidal system* and establish connections with the corpus striatum, red nucleus, substantia nigra, reticular formation, etc. (pp. 78 and 88).

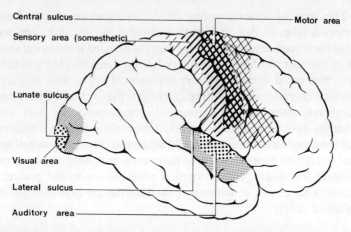

Fig. 30 The approximate cortical localization of motor, somatic sensory, auditory and visual functions on the lateral aspect of the cerebral hemisphere. The heavily shaded or stippled areas are the main afferent regions and the lighter adjacent zones are the so-called 'psychic' areas concerned with comparison and integration.

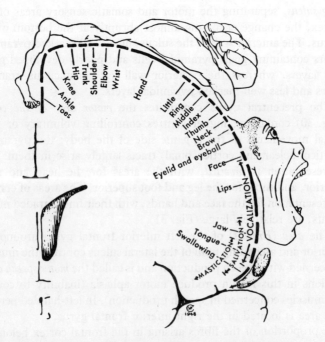

Fig. 31 Penfield's 'motor homunculus' shows the inverted representation of the body in the precentral gyrus and the disproportionate representation of various parts depending on their functional importance.

The non-motor parts of the frontal cortical areas used to be termed 'silent', because electrical stimulation of them evoked no response. They were regarded with great interest, however, because of their supposedly unusual degree of development in Man and the consequent belief that they were the seat of the 'mind'. But relatively the frontal lobes have undergone no more enlargement than the parietal or temporal lobes, so this erroneous supposition does not support the idea concerning the predominance of the frontal lobes in the highest mental processes, although it does not disprove their reputed role in the integration of these reactions and emotions that mould personality. They were also supposed to be specially important association areas, but the evidence does not suggest that they are more important in this respect than other lobes such as the parietal and temporal. There is thus no convincing anatomical basis for the belief that they are super-association areas or that they mastermind the activities of all other cortical areas.

There is evidence, however, of an intimate inter-relationship between the frontal lobes and the hypothalamus, with the anterior and medial thalamic nuclei acting as relay stations on the pathways between them. Thus fibres from cells in the hypothalamus form synapses around cells in the anterior and medial thalamic nuclei and the axons of the latter cells end mainly in the frontal and cingulate gyri (Fig. 32). Fibres from cells in these cortical areas project via relays in the same thalamic nuclei to the hypothalamus, brain stem and cord (Fig. 33). Thus afferent and efferent pathways exist linking these parts of the central nervous system. The hypothalamus assists in controlling visceral, vascular, rhythmic and other involuntary bodily activities which influence emotions and behaviour.

The efferents from the frontal lobes may be divided into five main groups:

1. *Pyramidal*. These are the corticonuclear and corticospinal motor pathways (p. 86).
2. *Corticothalamic* fibres pass from the frontal cortex to the medial and anterior thalamic nuclei. Fresh relays of fibres carry impulses to the hypothalamus (Fig. 33).
3. *Corticohypothalamic*. There are connections between the frontal cortex and hypothalamus via the thalamus, and there are some other direct connections (Fig. 33).
4. *Corticostriate*. These fibres terminate mainly in the caudate nucleus and constitute part of the extrapyramidal system (pp. 80 and 88).
5. *Frontopontine* fibres end round cells in the medial groups of pon-

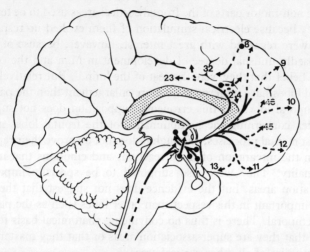

Fig. 32 Nervous pathways passing from the hypothalamus, mostly via relays in the thalamus, to frontal cortical areas and the cingulate gyrus.

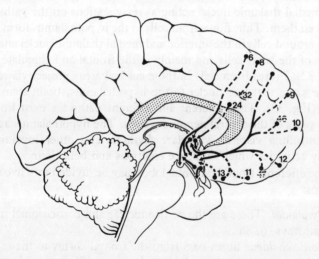

Fig. 33 Nervous pathways passing from frontal cortical areas and the cingulate gyrus, mostly via relays in the thalamus, to the hypothalamus.

tine nuclei (p. 36); they originate mainly in the middle and inferior frontal gyri.

Summary. The frontal lobes contain the higher centres for voluntary motor activities, they are closely interconnected with the hypothalamus and thalamus, and they may act as association areas correlating sensory impressions of various kinds with visceral activities. Lesions involving them produce motor and autonomic disturbances, alterations in behaviour and character, and diminish the ability to feel or notice certain types of pain.

The parietal lobes
The postcentral gyri are concerned with the reception and appreciation of *somatic sensory impulses* (Fig. 30), although, just as certain motor fibres arise in the postcentral cortex, so some sensory fibres end in precentral cortical areas. The sensory representation, like the motor, is crossed and inverted; and very sensitive parts such as the lips and finger-tips have disproportionately large cortical areas of representation (Fig. 34). The afferents concerned are the projections of the medial, spinal and trigeminal lemnisci, the fibres of which relay in the lateral thalamic nucleus *en route* to the cortex (pp. 90–94).

The parietal lobe is also an important association area and in it various somatic sensations are compared with previous similar impressions and with other sensations, e.g. from the adjacent visual

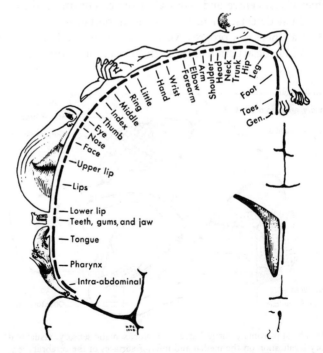

Fig. 34 Penfield's 'sensory homunculus' shows the inverted representation of the body in the postcentral gyrus and the disproportionate representation of various parts depending on their functional importance.

and auditory cortical centres. The position of the parietal lobes between the somatic sensory, visual and auditory cortical areas facilitates such co-ordination and permits refinements in interpretation such as the accurate perception of shape, size and texture. Lesions in this area of the brain produce disturbance or loss of these functions (agnosia), coupled with difficulties in talking and writing (sensory aphasia), particularly if the left inferior parietal lobule is affected.

The occipital lobes

The occipital cortex contains the *visuosensory and visuopsychic areas*, the so-called *higher visual centres* (Figs. 30 and 35). These provide an excellent example of the principle that in evolution anatomical connections and representation tend to shift from lower to higher centres in the brain. In fish and amphibia the highest visual centres are apparently confined to the midbrain tectum and there is no cortical visual representation. In reptiles and birds some degree of visual projection to the cerebral cortex exists, but the midbrain remains the chief visual centre and removal of the cerebrum produces only minor visual defects. In mammals the importance of the cortical visual areas increases progressively as the animal scale is ascended, so that in Man destruction of the cortical visual areas produces blind-

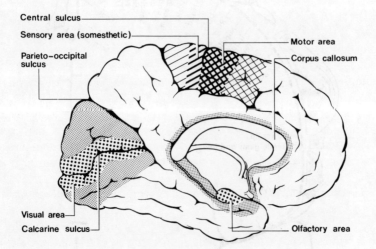

Fig. 35 The approximate cortical areas of motor, somatic sensory, visual and olfactory localization on the medial and inferior surfaces of the cerebral hemisphere. The heavily shaded or stippled areas are the main afferent or efferent regions and the lighter adjacent zones are 'psychic' areas concerned with comparison and integration.

ness, although pupillary reactions to light persist because they are mediated through the tectum, or rather the pretectum, which is the narrow zone between the cranial colliculi and thalami.

The *visual or striate area* (characterized by the presence throughout its extent of a thin white stria) is confined mainly to the walls of the calcarine sulcus, but also extends on to the surfaces of the cuneus above and the lingual gyrus below. On the lateral surface it is limited by the lunate sulcus. The fibres ending in these areas are the optic radiations from the lateral geniculate bodies, the *lower visual centres*. There is a definite relationship between each part of the retina, lateral geniculate body and striate area. Thus relatively large areas nearer the occipital poles are primarily concerned with impulses from the maculae and the peripheral parts of the retinae are represented further forward.

Visual impulses are received and decoded in the visual or visuo-sensory (visual or striate) areas, but the analysis and interpretation of these is effected in the adjacent visuopsychic areas of the occipital cortex.

The temporal lobes

These contain the higher *auditory* and *olfactory* centres, many association fibres (p. 82) end in them, they are the source of the temporopontine fibres (pp. 40, 85), but otherwise relatively little is known about their exact connections and functions as compared with those of the frontal lobes.

The auditory area of the cortex (Fig. 30) can be subdivided into an auditosensory zone in which the auditory radiations end, with an adjoining auditopsychic area. The auditosensory area occupies the middle part of the lower wall of the posterior ramus of the lateral sulcus, the transverse temporal (interlocking) gyri which cross it, and the adjacent part of the superior temporal gyrus. It is in this cortical area that sounds reach consciousness, although the analysis of their character, significance and direction is a function of the adjoining auditopsychic area which occupies most of the remainder of the superior temporal gyrus.

Giddiness and the sensations associated with alterations of balance are probably appreciated in the temporal cortex in areas contiguous to the higher auditory centres. Impulses originating in the vestibule and semicircular canals of the internal ear may be conveyed to these areas.

The higher olfactory areas are located in the uncus of the para-hippocampal gyrus (Fig. 35), a part of the rhinencephalon (see next section).

The rhinencephalon

This comprises all the parts concerned with the sensations of smell. In primitive animals this part of the brain overshadows all others, but in the higher vertebrates, and especially in Man, it has become reduced both in size and importance. Man is therefore, classified as microsmatic, whereas animals with highly developed olfactory functions are macrosmatic.

It includes the olfactory bulb and tract, rostral (anterior) perforated substance, piriform area, hippocampal formation, fornix and habenular region (habenula).

The **olfactory bulb** (Fig. 36) is a small ovoid structure which lies in the anterior end of the olfactory sulcus on the orbital surface of the frontal lobe. The delicate olfactory nerves enter its inferior surface. The *olfactory tract* is a slender band which passes backwards from the bulb and lies in the posterior end of the olfactory sulcus. The tract divides into medial and lateral *striae* posteriorly. The lateral stria ends in the uncus. The medial stria ascends anterior to the lamina terminalis and fades away in the adjacent parolfactory area of the frontal lobe below the rostrum (Fig. 25).

The **rostral (anterior) perforated substance** (Fig. 26) lies between the optic tract and the uncus, behind the diverging striae

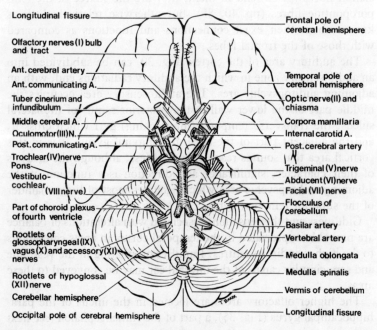

Longitudinal fissure

Olfactory nerves (I) bulb and tract

Ant. cerebral artery

Ant. communicating A.

Tuber cinerium and infundibulum

Middle cerebral A.

Oculomotor (III) N.

Post. communicating A.

Trochlear (IV) nerve

Pons

Vestibulo-cochlear (VIII nerve)

Part of choroid plexus of fourth ventricle

Rootlets of glossopharyngeal (IX) vagus (X) and accessory (XI) nerves

Rootlets of hypoglossal (XII) nerve

Cerebellar hemisphere

Occipital pole of cerebral hemisphere

Frontal pole of cerebral hemisphere

Temporal pole of cerebral hemisphere

Optic nerve (II) and chiasma

Corpora mamillaria

Internal carotid A.

Post. cerebral artery

Trigeminal (V) nerve

Abducent (VI) nerve

Facial (VII) nerve

Flocculus of cerebellum

Basilar artery

Vertebral artery

Medulla oblongata

Medulla spinalis

Vermis of cerebellum

Longitudinal fissure

Fig. 36 The inferior or basal surface of the brain.

of the olfactory tract. It is pierced by central branches of the anterior and middle cerebral arteries.

The **piriform area** includes the anterior part of the parahippocampal gyrus, the uncus and the anterior part of the dentate gyrus. The majority of the olfactory fibres end in the anterior part of the uncus which is the chief cortical *olfactory area*. By analogy with other special sensory zones it might be imagined that the remainder of the piriform area would be olfactopsychic in nature, but experimental investigations apparently do not support this.

The **hippocampal formation** is formed by the hippocampus and the posterior part of the dentate gyrus, together with a thin layer of grey matter (the *indusium griseum*) and strands of white fibres (the longitudinal striae, p. 54) which lie on the upper surface of the corpus callosum. The *hippocampus* is a curved eminence, about 5 cm long, which lies in the floor of the inferior horn of the lateral ventricle. It consists of grey matter, covered with a thin layer of white matter, the *alveus*. Its anterior end is somewhat enlarged and grooved; it resembles an animal's paw and so it is termed the *pes hippocampi*. The *dentate gyrus* is a crenated fringe of cortex lying between the parahippocampal gyrus and the fimbria hippocampi.

In Man few olfactory fibres end directly in the hippocampus, and although it may be partly concerned with olfaction, it may help in controlling visceral functions and emotional responses through its connections with the hypothalamus and via the latter and the thalamus with the frontal lobes.

The rhinencephalon is relatively rudimentary in Man, yet some parts included in it, such as the hippocampus and fornix, are better developed in humans than in macrosmatic animals. This indicates that their functions in Man are far from being purely olfactory. Some parts are concerned with autonomic and emotional activities.

The **fornix** is a bilateral C-shaped arrangement of white fibres which carry efferents from the hippocampi to the hypothalamus and commissural fibres between the right and left hippocampi.

The axons of the cells of the hippocampus form the *alveus*, the thin white layer on its ventricular surface, and they converge towards its medial edge to form a flattened band, the *fimbria hippocampi*, which lies immediately above the narrow dentate gyrus. In front the fimbria extends as far forwards as the uncus. Behind it runs upwards posterior to the thalamus, beneath the splenium of the corpus callosum, and then turns forwards above the thalamus; at this stage it forms the *crus of the fornix*. The two crura approach each other, lying below the corpus callosum, and are interconnected by a number of transverse strands which constitute the *commissure of the fornix.* Just in front of this the two crura lie in close apposition in the median plane and form the *body of the fornix*, which rests on the tela choroidea of the third ventricle (Fig. 37) and the medial part of the upper surface of the thalamus. The body is attached above to the under aspect of the corpus callosum and to the lower margin of the septum pellucidum; it helps to bound the choroidal fissure (p. 81) through which the pia mater of the tela choroidea becomes invaginated into the lateral ventricle.

Above the interventricular foramina the two halves of the body separate and form the two *columns of the fornix*, which curve down and back in front of the interventricular foramina and behind the anterior commissure. As they descend, each column inclines backwards and sinks into the anterior part of the homolateral wall of the third ventricle to end in the homolateral corpus mamillare. The fibres ending in the corpus mamillare form synapses with cells whose axons pass upwards in the mamillothalamic fasciculus to the anterior nucleus of the thalamus (Fig. 32).

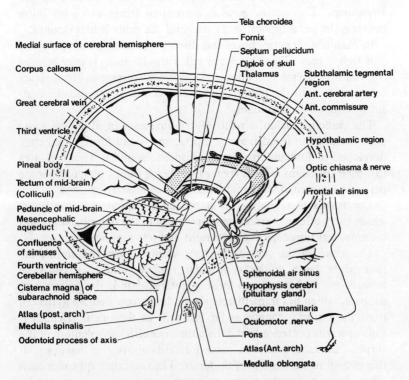

Fig. 37 A median sagittal section through the head. The falx cerebri has been removed to show the medial surface of the left cerebral hemisphere.

The **habenular region** or **habenula** (sometimes described as part of the diencephalon) includes the habenular nucleus which underlies the trigonum habenulae, the small depressed area on each side between the posterior part of the thalamus, the cranial colliculus and the stalk of the pineal body. Afferent fibres are conveyed to it in the *stria medullaris thalami*, a fine strand of fibres lying along the junction of the superior and medial surfaces of the thalamus, and efferent fibres pass in the fasciculus retroflexus (tractus habenulo-interpeduncularis) to the nucleus interpeduncularis in the interpeduncular (posterior) perforated substance. The two habenular nuclei are interconnected by the small *habenular commissure* which passes transversely above the stalk of the pineal body. The ependymal roof of the third ventricle is attached on each side along the line of the stria medullaris thalami.

The diencephalon
This is the part of the forebrain interposed between it and the midbrain, and it gives origin to important structures such as the:

Thalami
Medial and lateral geniculate bodies
Pineal body and habenula
Hypothalamus

The **thalami** (Figs. 38 and 39) are two large nuclear masses which in primitive vertebrates act as centres for the reception and correlation of sensory impressions and so greatly influence the reactions and behaviour of the animals. In more advanced types, as a result of the development of higher centres in the cerebral hemispheres, the thalami lose their ancient dominance, but they remain as important relay centres on the sensory pathways to the cortex.

They are ovoid in shape, about 4 cm in length, and are situated on each side of the third ventricle. Posteriorly they project backwards for some distance behind this cavity. Each thalamus has two ends and four surfaces.

The *anterior end* is smaller than the posterior and lies behind the interventricular foramen which connects the lateral and third ventricles.

The *posterior end* is large and prominent, forming a rounded projection termed the *pulvinar*, which partially overlies the cranial colliculus and cranial brachium of the same side.

The *superior surface* is not clearly demaracated from the lateral surface, but the line of junction between it and the medial surface is indicated by the *stria medullaris thalami*. It is separated from the

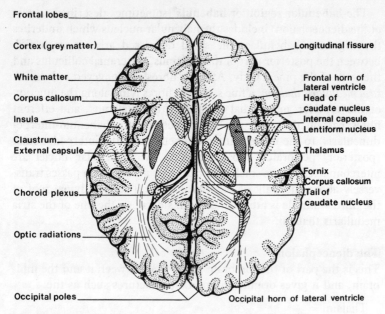

Frontal lobes

Cortex (grey matter)

White matter

Corpus callosum

Insula

Claustrum
External capsule

Choroid plexus

Optic radiations

Occipital poles

Longitudinal fissure

Frontal horn of
lateral ventricle
Head of
caudate nucleus
Internal capsule
Lentiform nucleus

Thalamus

Fornix
Corpus callosum
Tail of
caudate nucleus

Occipital horn of lateral ventricle

Fig. 38 Horizontal sections through the cerebral hemispheres. The section on the right side has been made about 1.25 cm above that on the left side.

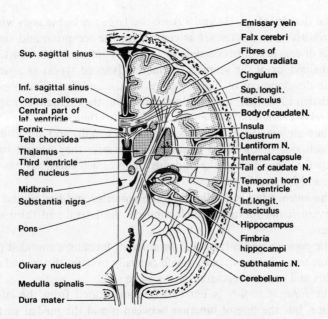

Sup. sagittal sinus

Inf. sagittal sinus
Corpus callosum
Central part of
lat. ventricle
Fornix
Tela choroidea
Thalamus
Third ventricle
Red nucleus
Midbrain
Substantia nigra
Pons

Olivary nucleus

Medulla spinalis
Dura mater

Emissary vein
Falx cerebri
Fibres of
corona radiata
Cingulum
Sup. longit.
fasciculus
Body of caudate N.
Insula
Claustrum
Lentiform N.
Internal capsule
Tail of caudate N.
Temporal horn of
lat. ventricle
Inf. longit.
fasciculus
Hippocampus
Fimbria
hippocampi
Subthalamic N.
Cerebellum

Fig. 39 Coronal section of half the head with the brain *in situ*.

ventricular surface of the caudate nucleus by a white strand, the *stria terminalis*, and also by the thalamostriate vein. The superior surface is divided into two areas by a faint groove which is an impression produced by the lateral margin of the fornix. The lateral area forms part of the floor of the central part of the lateral ventricle. The median area is covered by a double fold of pia mater called the tela choroidea of the third ventricle.

The *inferior surface* lies upon the upward prolongation of the tegmentum of the midbrain, the subthalamic tegmental region.

The *medial surface* forms part of the lateral wall of the third ventricle and is separated by a narrow interval from the corresponding surface of the opposite thalamus. The two thalami are connected in this region by a short flattened band, the *interthalamic adhesion*, which bridges across the cavity of the third ventricle.

The *lateral surface* is separated from the lentiform nucleus by the posterior limb of the *internal capsule*. Multiple fibres stream out from this surface and enter the internal capsule en route for the cerebral cortex. They form the *thalamic radiations*, which form a stratum on its lateral surface termed the *external medullary lamina*.

Structure and connections of the thalamus
Each thalamus consists mainly of grey matter, but its superior and lateral surfaces are covered by thin layers of white matter termed respectively the *stratum zonale* and the *external medullary lamina*. The grey matter is incompletely divided into anterior, medial and ventrolateral nuclei by a Y-shaped lamina of white matter termed the *internal medullary lamina*. The anterior and medial nuclei are both much smaller than the ventrolateral nucleus which lies between the external and internal medullary laminae. These three nuclei have been subdivided into many subsidiary nuclei whose individual connections and functions in Man, and even in animals, are still controversial, so here attention is confined to the main nuclei as most workers agree about their general connections. However some of these subdivisions, such as the thalamic intralaminar and reticular nuclei merit attention (p. 42).

The thalamus is the most important relay station on the somatic sensory pathways. It also acts as a centre for integrating impulses from many sources (somatic sensory, visual, visceral, cerebellar, etc.) before passing them on to the cerebral cortex. More primitive sensations, such as certain types of pain, may reach consciousness at this level and may still be appreciated when all connections between the thalamus and cortex are destroyed.

The connections are more readily understood if one studies the evolution of the thalamus. It has reached its definitive form by a process of accretion at successive stages of evolution, just as an historic building often consists of an agglomeration of structures of different periods. In lowly animals with relatively simple bodies no elaborate sensorium is necessary and the cortex is practically non-existent. In these the thalamus is represented by a few small nuclei. As the body increases in size and complexity the ordinary and special sensory mechanisms become increasingly important. This is associated with a proportionate increase in the thalamus and by the development of cortical areas connected anatomically and functionally with it. Thus the oldest parts of the cortex were probably developed as afferent projection areas connected with autonomic, olfactory and balancing or postural sensations, and other parts of the cortex, e.g. those associated with vision, hearing, memory, emotions, etc., evolved at later periods. The older parts of the thalamus are mainly represented in the human brain by the anterior and medial nuclei, but in the process of evolution they have undergone modification and further differentiation and their functions do not coincide exactly with the more primitive pattern, they have extensive connections with various areas of the cortex, especially in the frontal lobes and cingulate gyrus, and with other parts such as the hypothalamus and corpus striatum.

As evolution continued the cerebral cortex became still more extensive, and the thalamus also increased in size, mainly ventrolaterally and posteriorly, to form the large ventrolateral nucleus.

The anterior and medial thalamic nuclei act as relay stations on two-way corticohypothalamic pathways (Figs. 32 and 33). The ventrolateral nucleus acts as a relay station for the fibres in the medial, spinal and trigeminal lemnisci, and the fresh relays of fibres pass through the posterior limb of the internal capsule before radiating to the postcentral sensory cortex: some fibres from the heterolateral cerebellar dentate nucleus form synapses in its anterior part with neurons which have their terminations in the precentral motor cortex and adjacent areas in the frontal gyri. The posterior parts of the ventrolateral nucleus (including the pulvinar) are well developed only in the higher primates and they are interconnected with some other parts of the thalamus and with the parietal cortical areas.

Summary. The thalamus receives afferents from:

1. The medial, spinal and trigeminal lemnisci.
2. The hypothalamus (the mamillothalamic fasciculus, periventricular fibres, etc).
3. The corpus striatum.

4. The heterolateral dentate nucleus via the superior cerebellar peduncle.
5. The homolateral red nucleus, the reticular nuclei and other nuclei in the brain stem.
6. Most parts of the cerebral cortex.

The efferents proceed to:

1. Most parts of the cerebral cortex.
2. The hypothalamus.
3. The corpus striatum.
4. The brain stem and spinal cord.

The **geniculate bodies** are two small elevations on each side closely related to the thalami.

Each *medial geniculate body* is ovoid and lies beneath the homolateral pulvinar and lateral to the cranial colliculus. It is a relay station on the auditory pathway and receives fibres through the lateral lemniscus; a fresh relay of fibres carries the impulses to the temporal part of the cortex. The medial geniculate bodies are the *lower auditory centres*. They are connected by commissural fibres which pass through the medial roots of the optic tracts and through the posterior part of the optic chiasma. A low ridge, the *caudal brachium*, extends between the caudal collicus and the homolateral medial geniculate body.

Each *lateral geniculate body* is also ovoid and is situated on the undersurface of the pulvinar, anterior and lateral to the medial geniculate body. The *cranial brachium* connects it to the homolateral cranial colliculus. The majority of the visual fibres in the optic tract end in it and a fresh relay of fibres passes to the occipital part of the cortex. The lateral geniculate bodies are the chief lower visual centres.

The **pineal body** (epiphysis cerebri) is a small, cone-shaped, glandular structure which may pass its secretion into the third ventricle or into the blood. It lies in the depression between the cranial colliculi. It is attached in front by a short stalk to the *posterior (epithalamic)* and *habenular commissures*. It shows a tendency to fibrosis and calcification and when calcified it may readily be identified in radiographs.

The *posterior (epithalamic) commissure* is a fascicle of fibres which passes transversely above the upper end of the mesencephalic aqueduct; it helps to interconnect the cranial colliculi, the posterior parts of the thalami, and nuclei in opposite halves of the midbrain. Some of its fibres enter the medial longitudinal bundle.

The **habenula** was described on p. 68.

The **hypothalamus** (Fig. 37) is mainly derived from the diencephalon.

It comprises the:

Corpora mamillaria
Tuber cinereum and infundibulum
Neurohypophysis (post. lobe of pituitary)
The lateral wall of the third ventricle below and in front of the thalamus

The corpora mamillaria are two small hemispherical bodies lying side by side in front of the interpeduncular (posterior) perforated substance. Each contains a central grey core, surrounded by white matter derived mainly from the fibres of the homolateral column of the fornix. These fibres form synapses with the nerve cells in the grey core and a fresh relay of fibres passes partly to the anterior nucleus of the thalamus and partly to the tegmentum of the midbrain.

Tuber cinereum and *infundibulum*. The former is a small elevation of grey matter located in the midline between the optic chiasma in front and the corpora mamillaria behind. From its anterior part a conical process, the *infundibulum*, projects downwards to become continuous with the neurohypophysis (posterior lobe of pituitary); it is hollow in its upper part and contains a small prolongation of the cavity of the third ventricle.

The *hypophysis* (*pituitary gland*) (Fig. 16 and 37) is the most important of the endocrine glands and has been described as the conductor of the endocrine orchestra. It is an ovoid body (about 1.25 cm in its transverse and 0.8 cm in its anteroposterior diameter) which is attached to the end of the infundibulum and lies in the sella turcica of the sphenoid bone. Except above, the hypophysis is surrounded by venous sinuses – by the cavernous sinuses and their contained structures on each side, by the intercavernous sinuses in front and behind and by unnamed channels which lie beneath the gland and separate it from the body of the sphenoid bone and its contained air sinuses.

It consists of two lobes, a larger anterior and a smaller posterior, and they differ in their development and structure.

The *anterior lobe* (adenohypophysis) is derived from an ectodermal diverticulum of the primitive oral cavity and in the course of development this communication (the craniopharyngeal canal) is obliterated. It is incompletely divided into anterior and posterior parts by a cleft representing the remnant of the primitive cavity of the diverticulum. The anterior part is very vascular and bulges upwards around the infundibulum towards the tuber cinereum. The posterior part of the anterior lobe is smaller and less vascular and intervenes as a narrowish strip, the *pars intermedia*, between the anterior part of the anterior lobe and the true posterior lobe.

The *posterior lobe* (neurohypophysis) is smaller than the anterior. It is derived from a diverticulum which grows down from that part of the diencephalon which later forms the floor of the third ventricle. The original lumen disappears in Man except in the upper part of the infundibulum, but in some animals there is a persistent space in the posterior lobe which opens directly into the third ventricle. Despite its neurogenic origin this lobe contains few or no nerve cells, but it does contain a modified type of nervous or neuroglial tissue.

The considerable variety of cells in different parts of the hypophysis elaborate a number of hormones which play important but differing roles in the body. The intimate developmental and anatomical relationships with the hypothalamus are noteworthy: the hypophysis receives nerve fibres direct from the supraoptic and paraventricular hypothalamic nuclei (p. 100) and there are also close vascular connections. The proximity to the optic chiasma should be noted, since it explains the visual changes frequently associated with enlargements of the gland which produce pressure on adjacent structures.

The *optic chiasma* (Figs. 36 and 37) which lies at the junction of the anterior wall and floor of the third ventricle gives rise posteriorly to the optic tracts. Functionally it is *not* a part of the hypothalamus.

The *lateral walls of the third ventricle below and in front of the thalamus* are important parts of the hypothalamus. The division between the hypothalamus and the thalamus is indicated on each side by a slight curve groove, the *hypothalamic sulcus*, which extends from the interventricular foramen to the mesencephalic aqueduct. Several nuclei exist in the grey matter lining this area (Fig. 49); they are concerned with autonomic activities and some are closely connected with the hypophysis.

The hypothalamus is a complex neuroglandular mechanism concerned with the regulation of visceral and other activities. This is reiterated in the section on the autonomic part of the nervous system (p. 100).

The third ventricle
The third ventricle (Figs. 37 and 39) is a narrow median cleft which possesses a roof, anterior, posterior and two lateral walls.

The *roof* is the thin layer of ependyma stretching between the upper edges of the side walls. This layer is closely applied to the under aspect of a double fold of pia mater, the *tela choroidea of the third ventricle*, and the roof is invaginated into the cavity along its whole length by delicate vascular tufts of the pia mater arranged in two parallel rows; these are the *choroid plexuses* of the third ventricle.

The *floor* is formed from before backwards by the optic chiasma, the tuber cinereum and infundibulum, the corpora mamillaria, the posterior (interpeduncular) perforated substance and the uppermost part of the tegmentum of the midbrain. The cavity of the ventricle is prolonged downwards into the infundibulum as a small recess.

The *anterior wall* is formed by a delicate layer of grey and white matter, the *lamina terminalis*, which stretches between the optic chiasma and the rostrum of the corpus callosum; it represents the cephalic end of the primitive neural tube. In the upper part of the lamina, at the junction of the roof and anterior wall, is the *anterior* (rostral) *commissure*. It is a compact and rounded bundle in the midline, but its fibres diverge as they curve outwards, grooving the antero-inferior part of the corpus striatum. Many fibres connect the olfactory and piriform areas and others progress into the temporal lobes where they spread out like the frayed ends of a string to end in the cortex of the temporal poles. On each side, just posterior to this commissure, there is an *interventricular foramen* through which the lateral and third ventricles communicate. Each foramen is oval or crescentic in shape and lies between the anterior end of the thalamus and the curving column of the fornix.

The short *posterior wall* is formed by the base of the pineal body and the posterior (epithalamic) and habenular commissures.

Each *lateral wall* is formed above and behind by the anterior two-thirds of the medial surface of the thalamus and below and in front by part of the hypothalamus. These two areas are separated by the hypothalamic sulcus. The junction of the side wall and the roof corresponds with the line of the stria medullaris thalami. The columns of the fornix form the anterior margins of the interventricular foramina and then run downwards in the lateral walls towards the corpora mamillaria; they sink into the walls as they descend and so are most easily distinguished above. The interthalamic adhesion bridges across the narrow ventricular space.

The interpeduncular fossa

This lies between the diverging cerebral peduncles and contains the corpora mamillaria and the interpeduncular (posterior) perforated substance which transmits the posteromedial branches of the posterior cerebral arteries. The diverging peduncles are bridged across by arachnoid and the resulting cisterna interpeduncularis contains the posterior part of the arterial circle (p. 106).

The optic chiasma and optic tracts

The chiasma is a flattened mass of nerve fibres lying at the junction of the optic nerves and optic tracts (Figs. 36 and 37). The nerves are attached to its anterolateral and the tracts to its posterolateral angles and the arrangement resembles an X. It lies at the junction of the anterior wall and floor of the third ventricle, being attached to the lamina terminalis above and to the tuber cinereum behind, Laterally it is in relationship with the termination of the internal carotid artery. Below it rests on the sulcus prechiasmatis of the sphenoid bone, above and in front of the hypophysis cerebri.

Fibres originating in the retina travel back to the chiasma in the optic nerves. In the chiasma the medial fibres in the nerves, those coming from the nasal halves of the retinae, decussate and enter the opposite optic tract (Fig. 40). The fibres from the temporal sides of the retinae lie in the lateral parts of the optic nerves and chiasma and do not cross but continue backwards in the optic tract of the same side. The nasal and temporal fibres from the maculae behave in exactly the same way as the other retinal fibres and they occupy the central part of the chiasma.

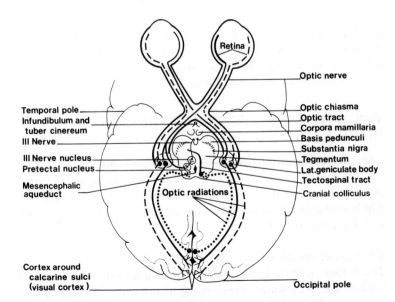

Fig. 40 The visual pathways. Other connections are shown which are concerned in visual reflexes of various types.

The *optic tracts* pass backwards and outwards from the chiasma, between the rostral perforated substance and the tuber cinereum. They then wind round and become adherent to the upper parts of the cerebral peduncles and divide into medial and lateral roots.

The medial root enters the *medial geniculate body*, but many or most of its fibres are derived from the opposite medial geniculate body via the optic tracts and chiasma and so are commissural (supraoptic commissures). Others passing to the caudal colliculus are *not* parts of the visual pathway.

The lateral root ends mainly in the *lateral geniculate body* which is the chief *lower visual centre*. Other fibres end in small pretectal nuclei in the vicinity of the cranial colliculi which are connected with the oculomotor nuclei and are concerned with pupillary reflexes. Still other fibres may pass to the pulvinar and cranial colliculi. The lateral root fibres convey visual sensations from the retina, and when they relay in the lateral geniculate body a new set of fibres arise which passes through the posterior part of the internal capsule and then by the optic radiations to the *higher visual centres* in the occipital cortex. A few efferent fibres pass forwards through the optic tracts, chiasma and nerves to the retina.

The fibres in the optic radiations are not all directed towards the cortex. Some pass from the higher cortical centres to the cranial colliculi, relay there, and are then conveyed by the tectobulbar and tectospinal tracts to the nuclei of the oculomotor, trochlear, abducent and accessory nerves and to ventral cornual cells in the cervical segments of the cord. These tracts convey impulses concerned with certain types of visual reflexes, particularly with the reflex movements of the head and eyes which occur in response to visual stimuli.

THE INTERNAL STRUCTURE OF THE CEREBRAL HEMISPHERES

Each cerebral hemisphere consists of a grey convoluted *cortex*, a central mass of *white matter* containing several *buried masses of grey matter* and a large irregular cavity, the *lateral ventricle* (Figs. 38 and 39). The buried grey matter comprises the corpus striatum, the claustrum and the amygdaloid body.

The corpus striatum

The corpus striatum is incompletely divided into the lentiform and caudate nuclei by white fibres passing to and from the cerebral cortex. These fibres also separate the corpus striatum from the nearby thalamus (Figs. 38, 39 and 44).

The caudate nucleus

This is of a curved piriform shape. Its rounded head projects into the floor of the frontal horn of the lateral ventricle. Laterally and below it is partially separated from the lentiform nucleus by a lamina of white matter, but bands of grey and white matter are commingled in this area and on section they have a *striated* appearance. Passing backwards the head rapidly tapers into a narrower body, which lies in the floor of the central part of the lateral ventricle on the lateral side of the thalamus. The body ends in a slender tail which curves downwards behind the thalamus and finally turns forwards in the roof of the temporal horn of the lateral ventricle to end in the *amygdaloid body*, an almond-shaped mass of grey matter situated in the forepart of the roof of the temporal horn.

A small bundle of white fibres, the *stria terminalis*, emerges from the posterior part of the amygdaloid body and runs backwards along the medial side of the caudate nucleus in the roof of the temporal horn of the lateral ventricle. It then turns upwards behind the thalamus, before running forwards in the groove between the central part of the caudate nucleus and the thalamus in the floor of the body of the lateral ventricle. Behind the interventricular foramen it bends downwards and ends by sending fibres to several nuclei in the hypothalamus and it may contribute some fibres to the rostral (anterior) commissure.

The lentiform nucleus

This is lens-shaped and the medial surface is more convex than the lateral. It is surrounded by white matter and so appears to be encapsulated. The thinner lamina of white matter on the outer side is termed the *external capsule* and it is bounded on its lateral surface by a narrow stratum of grey matter, the *claustrum*, which in turn is separated from the cortex of the insula by another thin white layer (Fig. 44). The thicker lamina of white matter on the inner side is the *internal capsule* which separates it from the head of the caudate nucleus in front and the thalamus behind. The inferior surface is grooved by the rostral (anterior) commissure as it sweeps outwards into the temporal lobe, and just anterior to this the lentiform nucleus is in contact with the rostral (anterior) perforated substance. On section the nucleus is seen to consist of a darker lateral portion, the *putamen*, and a smaller medial part, the *globus pallidus*.

The connections of the corpus striatum are intricate and are only partially known. Fibres from the frontal, temporal and parietal cortical areas and from the thalamus end in the putamen and caudate nucleus. These fibres form synapses with cells in these parts of the corpus striatum and fresh relays of fibres pass mainly to the globus pallidus; others pass to the thalamus and midbrain. Efferent fibres from the globus pallidus pass to the thalamus and hypothalamus, but the majority stream caudally to end in the red, reticular and subthalamic nuclei, and perhaps in the substantia nigra.

This complex arrangement of connections linking the cortex, the corpus striatum and brain stem influences various 'voluntary' motor activites and it is termed the *extrapyramidal system*. The red and reticular nuclei also have important cerebellar connections, and they influence lower centres in the brain stem and cord through *rubrobulbar, reticulobulbar, rubrospinal* and *reticulospinal tracts* originating in them. The rubrobulbar fibres end mainly in the olivary nuclei and from the latter *olivospinal* fibres descend to end around ventral cornual cells in the cord. The rubrospinal tracts in Man may end in the upper parts of the cord, but the reticular tracts descend to lower levels and also end around ventral and lateral cornual cells. These tracts may be both crossed and uncrossed and accompany the ventral and lateral corticospinal tracts but, unlike the latter, they are interrupted by a series of synapses.

The lateral ventricles

Each cerebral hemisphere is hollowed out by an irregular cavity, the lateral ventricle (Figs. 38 and 41). The two lateral ventricles communicate with the third ventricle through the *interventricular foramina*. Each consists of a central part and three horns (frontal or

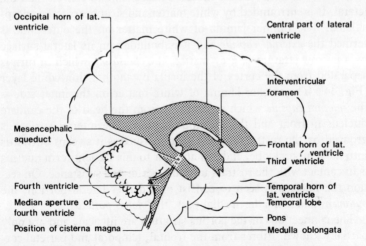

Occipital horn of lat. ventricle

Central part of lateral ventricle

Interventricular foramen

Mesencephalic aqueduct

Frontal horn of lat. ventricle

Third ventricle

Fourth ventricle

Temporal horn of lat. ventricle

Temporal lobe

Median aperture of fourth ventricle

Pons

Position of cisterna magna

Medulla oblongata

Fig. 41 This diagram shows the shape, extent and interconnections of the ventricles and their relative positions in the brain.

anterior, occipital or posterior and temporal or inferior), and all these communicate freely with the central part or body of the ventricle.

The *central part* is slightly curved, triangular on transverse section, and extends from the interventricular foramen to the splenium. The roof is formed by the under surface of the corpus callosum and the medial wall by the posterior part of the septum pellucidum. The floor is formed from the lateral to the medial side by the caudate nucleus, the stria terminalis, the lateral part of the upper surface of the thalamus, the choroid plexus and the lateral edge of the fornix (Fig. 39).

The *frontal horn* curves forwards and slightly outwards and downwards into the frontal lobe. It also is triangular in section and is bounded above by the corpus callosum and medially by the anterior part of the septum pellucidum. The floor is formed by the bulging head of the caudate nucleus. In front it ends blindly, its limit being the posterior surface of the genu of the corpus callosum.

The *occipital horn* passes backwards into the occipital lobe. It is triangular in section and its roof and lateral wall are formed by fibres of the corpus callosum. The fibres of the forceps occipitalis sweeping backwards to the occipital lobe produce a bulge in the upper part of the medial wall which is termed the *bulb of the occipital horn*, Beneath this there is a second elevation, the *calcar avis*, which corresponds to the deep groove produced by the calcarine sulcus. Posteriorly this horn tapers to a blind end where the walls unite.

The *temporal horn* curves downwards behind the thalamus and then passes forwards into the temporal lobe. It is longer than the other horns but, like them, it is triangular in section, with fibres of the corpus callosum forming its roof and lateral wall. The tail of the caudate nucleus, the stria terminalis and the amygdaloid body also lie in the roof. The floor is formed by the hippocampus, the fimbria hippocampi, the choroid plexus and the collateral eminence. The last is an elevation lying lateral to the hippocampus, which becomes triangular in shape posteriorly (the trigonum collaterale) at the junction of the temporal and occipital horns; it corresponds with the middle part of the collateral sulcus. The temporal horn ends blindly about 2.5 cm behind the temporal pole.

The choroidal fissure

This is cleft through which the pia mater invaginates the ependyma of the walls of the lateral ventricles to form the choroid plexuses of these ventricles. On each side it extends in an arched fashion from the interventricular foramen to the extremity of the temporal horn.

The fissure lies between the lateral edges of the fornix and the superior and posterior surfaces of the thalamus, and below it lies between the fimbria hippocampi and the tail of the caudate nucleus. It follows that the choroid plexuses of the lateral ventricles, which are formed by the invagination of fringed tufts of the vascular pia mater through this fissure, are also highly arched in their disposition.

The pia mater between the fornix and the thalamus forms a triangular shaped double layer, the *tela choroidea* of the third ventricle (Figs. 37 and 39) Its apex is in the region of the closely placed interventricular foramina. The base corresponds in level with the posterior surfaces of the thalami and here the two layers separate, the upper ascending over the back of the splenium to become continuous with the pia mater on its upper surface, and the lower descending to become continuous with the pia mater over the tectum of the midbrain. The choroid plexuses of the third ventricle depend from the under surface of this layer in the mid-line.

The white matter of the cerebral hemispheres
The white matter of the cerebral hemispheres consists of nerve fibres embedded in neuroglia and they may be classified as:
1. Commissural fibres interconnecting corresponding areas in the *opposite* hemispheres.
2. Association fibres interconnecting different cortical areas in the *same* hemisphere.
3. Itinerant or projection fibres connecting the cerebrum and cerebellum with the brain stem and the spinal cord and vice versa.

Commissural fibres
These include the corpus callosum, the anterior (rostral) and posterior (epithalamic) commissures, the hippocampal and habenular commissures and the supraoptic commissures connecting the medial geniculate bodies and caudal colliculi via the optic tracts and chiasma. All these have already been described.

Association fibres
These may be long (connecting distant gyri) or short (connecting adjacent gyri) (Figs. 42 and 43). The short fibres lie just beneath the cortex , but the long fibres lie more deeply and may be grouped into rather indefinite bundles, e.g. the *superior longitudinal fisciculus* which sweeps backwards from the frontal lobe to the occipital lobe and sends some fibres downwards into the posterior part of the temporal lobe; the *inferior longitudinal fasciculus* which runs between the

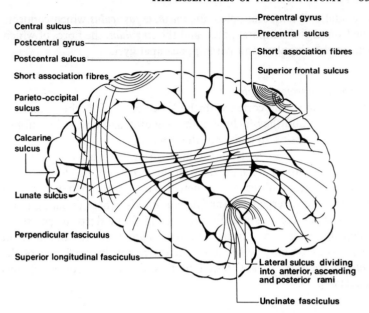

Fig. 42 Chief association tracts in cerebral hemisphere superimposed on an outline drawing of its superolateral surface.

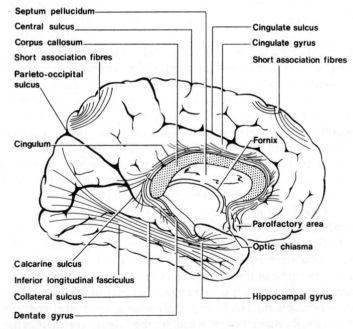

Fig. 43 Chief association tracts in cerebral hemisphere superimposed on an outline drawing of its medial and inferior surfaces.

occipital and temporal poles; the *uncinate fasciculus* which connects the frontal and temporal poles; and the *cingulum*, the fibres of which run in the cingulate and parahippocampal gyri.

Itinerant or projection fibres

These connect the cortex with the lower parts of the brain and the spinal cord and they include both ascending and descending fibres, i.e. fibres passing to and from the brain.

The itinerant fibres from the more primitive parts of the cortex, the hippocampus, are aggregated in the *fornix* (pp. 67–68).

The itinerant fibres of the newer parts of the cortex converge towards and diverge from the *internal capsule*. These radiating fibres intersect the commissural fibres, but mostly lie deep to the association fibres, and they form the *corona radiata*. Below, the fibres of the corona become concentrated in the relatively small area of the *internal capsule*, so any lesion in this situation produces serious effects.

The internal capsule

This is the lamina of white matter lying between the head of the caudate nucleus and the thalamus medially and the lentiform nucleus laterally (Figs. 38, 39 and 44). It is angulated to conform to the shape of the medial surface of the lentiform nucleus and consists of anterior and posterior limbs, with an intervening *genu*. This arrangement is appreciated most easily if horizontal sections of the hemisphere are examined. The *anterior limb* has the head of the caudate nucleus on its medial side and the lentiform nucleus laterally and the longer *posterior limb* is interposed between the thalamus medially and the lentiform nucleus laterally. The thalamus extends further back than the lentiform nucleus (Fig. 44) and so the most posterior part of the internal capsule is *retrolentiform*. Above the fibres of the internal capsule are directly continuous with those of the corona radiata. Below they are directly continuous with the descending fibres in the bases of the cerebral peduncles and the ascending fibres in the tegmentum of the midbrain.

The fibres in the internal capsule are arranged in a definite order. The anterior limb contains frontopontine and thalamocortical fibres. The former arise in the frontal cortex and end in the nuclei pontis, where fresh relays of fibres commence and pass to the opposite cerebellar hemisphere. The latter mainly arise in the medial and anterior thalamic nuclei and proceed to the frontal cortex. Corticothalamic fibres pass in the opposite direction.

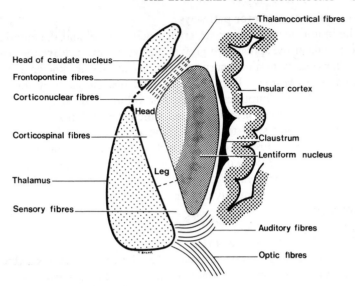

Fig. 44 A horizontal section of the internal capsule, showing the location of the chief groups of nerve fibres.

The genu and anterior half or two-thirds of the posterior limb contain the pyramidal fibres of the great somatic motor pathways. These fibres arise mainly in the precentral gyrus and pass downwards to the brain stem and spinal cord. Those in the genu (corticonuclear fibres) carry impulses for the muscles at the head end of the body and those for the trunk and extremities are arranged in order from before backwards in the posterior limb (corticospinal fibres).

The remainder of the posterior limb is occupied mainly by general and special sensory fibres. The posterior half or one-third of the posterior limb is occupied by thalamocortical fibres which arise in the lateral thalamic nucleus and ascend to the postcentral gyrus; they are part of the great somatic sensory pathways. Temporopontine and parietopontine fibres descend through this part of the posterior limb. The retrolentiform area contains fibres of the auditory radiation which arise in the medial geniculate body and fibres of the optic radiation which arise in the lateral geniculate body, and these pass respectively to the temporal and occipital parts of the cortex.

THE CHIEF NERVE TRACTS

The chief tracts connecting the brain and spinal cord are grouped as (1) motor, (2) sensory, (3) cerebellar and (4) autonomic.

The efferent or motor pathways

The motor neurons in certain cranial nerve nuclei and the anterior horn cells of the spinal cord grey matter whose axons leave the central nervous system to innervate voluntary muscle are known as the *lower motor neurons*. They form the *final common pathway* for the passage of nerve impulses to striated or voluntary muscle.

The *upper motor neuron* systems which descend from the cerebrum and brain stem to influence the activity of the lower motor neurons, either directly or through short intermediate neurons (interneurons), include two closely associated groups of fibres on each side, namely the *pyramidal* and the *extrapyramidal tracts*. Both of these tracts are intimately concerned with the control of voluntary movements.

The pyramidal tracts (Fig. 45)

These are long pathways originating in the cerebral cortex, which descend to terminate in certain cranial nerve nuclei (corticonuclear fibres) or in the anterior grey columns of the spinal cord (corticospinal fibres).

Each tract contains around one million fibres and the majority arise from neurons in the motor cortex (precentral gyrus) and adjacent posterior ends of frontal gyri. The remainder may come from other cortical areas or the corpus striatum, and a small number may be proprioceptive fibres ending in the postcentral gyrus. Incidentally, only a minority of the fibres are axons of the giant pyramidal cells typically seen in the motor cortex. *The tracts derive their name from the fact that they form the pyramids of the medulla oblongata.*

The pyramidal fibres converge through the corona radiata to the internal capsule where they occupy the genu and anterior half or two-thirds of the posterior limb (Fig. 44). Within the internal capsule there is an orderly arrangement of the fibres; the corticonuclear fibres destined to form synapses within certain cranial nerve nuclei occupy the genu, while the corticospinal fibres for the neck, upper limb, trunk and lower limb, are situated in sequence in the posterior limb. These fibres then descend in the middle three-fifths of the basis pedunculi of the midbrain , the corticonuclear fibres being placed medially while the lower limb fibres of the corticospinal tract are mostly situated laterally.

Most of the corticonuclear (geniculate) fibres cross the midline in succession in the brain stem to end in the motor nuclei of the cranial nerves controlling ocular, masticatory, facial, laryngeal, pharyngeal and lingual musculature. However, it should be noted that some

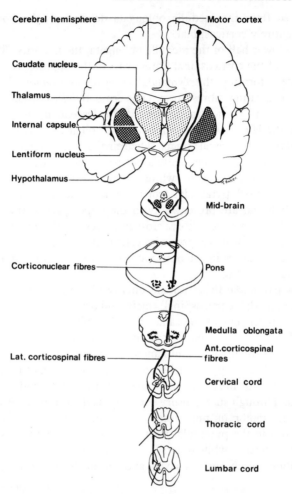

Cerebral hemisphere

Motor cortex

Caudate nucleus

Thalamus

Internal capsule

Lentiform nucleus

Hypothalamus

Mid-brain

Corticonuclear fibres

Pons

Medulla oblongata

Ant. corticospinal fibres

Lat. corticospinal fibres

Cervical cord

Thoracic cord

Lumbar cord

Fig. 45 The pyramidal tracts: the chief efferent pathways from the cortex to the voluntary motor nuclei of the brain stem (corticonuclear fibres) and to the ventral cornual cells of the spinal cord (corticospinal tracts).

corticonuclear fibres remain *uncrossed* and arborize in relation to ipsilateral lower motor neurons.

The pyramidal fibres continue their descent through the pons where they are separated into several small bundles by the transversely disposed ponticerebellar fibres. Below the pons the fibres are closely grouped together in the pyramids on the ventral aspect of the medulla oblongata. By this level most of the corticonuclear fibres have already decussated to end in the above-mentioned cranial nerve nuclei, so from the medulla oblongata downwards the fibres are almost entirely corticospinal.

In the lower half of the medulla oblongata, the majority (85 to 90 per cent) of the corticospinal fibres cross to the opposite side of the brain stem forming the *pyramidal or motor decussation* (Fig. 19). These decussating fibres form criss-cross bundles which incline backwards and then turn downwards to descend in the posterior parts of the lateral white columns of the spinal cord as the lateral pyramidal (corticospinal) tracts. The remainder of the corticospinal fibres do not cross in the medulla but pass downwards on the same side in the ventral (anterior) white columns of the spinal cord as the ventral (anterior) pyramidal (corticospinal) tracts; these are relatively small and are present only in the upper part of the cord as most of their constituent fibres cross in succession through the white commissure to form synapses with cells in the ventral (anterior) column of grey matter in the opposite side of the cervical segments of the spinal cord (Fig. 45).

A few pyramidal fibres remain uncrossed, descend in the homolateral pyramidal (corticospinal) tracts, and terminate around ventral (anterior) horn cells of the same side. Possibly these fibres help in controlling muscles such as the intercostals and diaphragm that normally act equally and simultaneously on both sides.

Incidentally, the pyramidal tracts are not entirely motor; some of their constituent fibres or their collaterals may end around sensory neurons. Through such sensory connections the cerebral cortex may modify its motor output. Some other fibres ascending from the spinal cord in the pyramidal tracts form synapses with cells in the brain stem nuclei, while others, which may be concerned with proprioception, reach cortical levels and terminate in the postcentral gyrus.

The extrapyramidal system
This term is applied to a complex series of tracts interconnecting various areas of the cerebral cortex (including the motor areas), the subcortical nuclei of the corpus striatum, and several important brain stem nuclei – substantia nigra, red nucleus, olivary nucleus and reticular nuclei. From some of these nuclei, which are also strongly influenced by other areas of the brain and notably the cerebellum, tracts descend to lower levels of the brain stem and spinal cord to influence lower motor neurons through intermediary neurons.

The main descending extrapyramidal tracts to the lower brain stem are the rubrobulbar (which end mainly in the olivary nuclei) and reticulobulbar tracts from the red nuclei and reticular nuclei respectively. Rubrospinal, reticulospinal and olivospinal tracts, both crossed and uncrossed, accompany the ventral (anterior) and lateral pyramidal (corticospinal) tracts (Fig. 46) to terminate in relationship to interneurons in the ventral (anterior) and lateral grey columns of the spinal cord. In humans the rubrospinal tract extends only into the upper part of the spinal cord; below this level the influence of the red nuclei is probably conducted along descending reticulospinal pathways.

The pyramidal and extrapyramidal systems ultimately produce their effects through the same final common pathways, namely the lower motor neurons, which are also influenced reflexly by sensory impulses received through cranial and spinal nerves. Voluntary movements, therefore, are under the control of both these motor systems. The pyramidal (corticospinal) tracts are principally concerned with precise or skilled voluntary movements of the more distal parts of the limbs. The extrapyramidal system is concerned with the regulation of muscle tone and thus influences postural activities and the more stereotyped movements.

The influence of the extrapyramidal system is chiefly inhibitory. Thus lesions of the subcortical and midbrain nuclei associated with

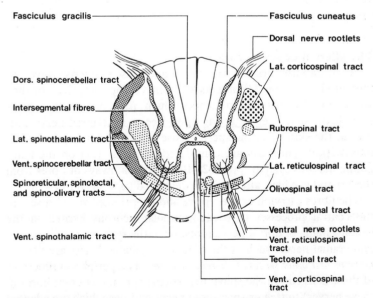

Fig. 46 A transverse section of the spinal cord showing the positions of the chief ascending (afferent) and descending (efferent) nerve tracts. The locations of these tracts vary to some extent at different levels.

this system may result in exaggerated postural tonus, hypertonicity or spasticity of voluntary muscles, and uncontrolled tremors or movements. Lesions of the pyramidal fibres above their decussation produce a heterolateral (contralateral) paralysis of voluntary muscles to a varying extent. Thus damage to the corticospinal fibres leads to an impairment of voluntary movement, especially of the precise movements of the distal parts of the limbs and their digits. The effects on muscles supplied by the cranial nerves will depend on the site of the lesion(s) with respect to the decussation of the corticonuclear fibres and whether or not the muscles and movements involved are represented bilaterally in the cerebral cortex.

The tectospinal and vestibulospinal tracts
These are two other descending pathways which also influence motor activities. The former originate in the colliculi and the fibres descend to arborize around cells in the *opposite* cranial nerve nuclei or in the ventral (anterior) grey columns of the cord. The vestibulospinal tract arises in the lateral vestibular nucleus and its fibres descend to terminate around cells in the ventral (anterior) grey column of the *same* side. The tectal and vestibular tracts bring the ventral horn cells under the influence of the colliculi and vestibular nuclei and modify their activities in accordance with stimuli received from the eyes and ears.

The afferent or sensory tracts
Afferent impulses arise in the viscera and vessels (interoceptive); in the muscles, tendons, ligaments and joints (proprioceptive); or they are produced by external influences (touch, pain, temperature, pressure, light, sound, etc.), acting upon free or specialised nerve endings in the skin or in the special sense organs (exteroceptive). The interoceptive pathways are considered in the section on the autonomic nervous system (pp. 102–103). The pathways of fibres from the ear and eye have already been described (pp. 38 and 77–78).

The fibres carrying exteroceptive and proprioceptive impulses are the central processes of pseduo-unipolar neurons located in the spinal ganglia of dorsal nerve roots, or in the sensory ganglia of certain cranial nerves such as the trigeminal ganglia. These are the *primary or first order sensory (afferent) neurons*. The peripheral processes of these cells run in the spinal nerves (they are the afferent fibres in these nerves) to free or specialised nerve endings which are adapted to respond to different types of stimuli (see Fig. 8). The central processes of the pseudo-unipolar neurons, which convey the afferent impulses subserving the various sensory modalities into the spinal cord, may terminate in various ways.

A small proportion of the dorsal root fibres on entering the spinal cord pass directly to arborize around motor neurons in the ventral (anterior) horn of the grey matter, forming monosynaptic reflex arcs. Others synapse with cells in the dorsal (posterior) horn of grey matter, which then influence ventral horn cells via reflex arcs involving two or more neurons (Fig. 7). The majority form synapses with dorsal horn cells, with cells in the thoracic nucleus at the base of the dorsal horn of spinal cord grey matter, or with the nucleus gracilis

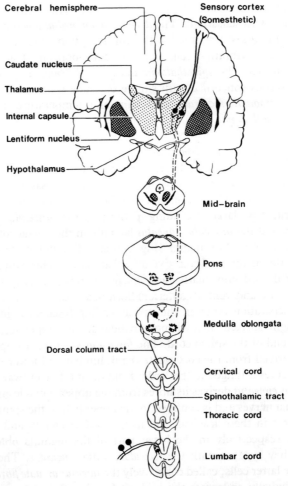

Cerebral hemisphere
Sensory cortex (Somesthetic)
Caudate nucleus
Thalamus
Internal capsule
Lentiform nucleus
Hypothalamus
Mid-brain
Pons
Medulla oblongata
Dorsal column tract
Cervical cord
Spinothalamic tract
Thoracic cord
Lumbar cord

Fig. 47 The chief somatic afferent pathways conveying somatic sensory impulses upwards to the cortex.

and nucleus cuneatus; these cells and their processes are the *secondary or second order sensory neurons*.

Many of the secondary sensory neurons transmit afferent impulses which will ultimately give rise to sensations appreciated at a conscious level, and they *cross* to the opposite side in the spinal cord or brain stem and proceed to the ventrolateral nuclei of the thalamus. Here the axons of these neurons synapse with the *tertiary or third order sensory neurons* in these thalamic nuclei. A fresh relay of fibres from these cells then pass through the posterior limb of the internal capsule (Fig. 44) and the corona radiata to the main somatic sensory area in the postcentral gyrus of the cerebral cortex (Fig. 30).

In the spinal cord and brain stem there are two major tract systems concerned with sensations. The *dorsal column/medial lemniscal system* conveys impulses concerned with proprioception, fine or discriminative touch, vibration sensation and a proportion of autonomic afferent fibres. The *spinothalamic tracts/spinal lemniscal system* conveys impulses concerned with simple or crude touch and pressure (*ventral spinothalamic tract*) and pain and temperature sensation (*lateral spinothalamic tract*).

Dorsal column – medial lemniscal system
The dorsal root afferent fibres concerned with conscious proprioception, fine or discriminative touch, vibration sensation and some autonomic sensory fibres, on entering the spinal cord turn upwards and form two large ascending pathways, the *fasciculus gracilis* medially and the *fasciculus cuneatus* laterally in the dorsal column of the spinal cord white matter (Figs. 46 and 47). Before turning to ascend, the incoming fibres give off collateral branches which enter the spinal cord grey matter and engage in reflex activity through intermediate and ventral (anterior) horn neurons.

The separation between the two ascending fasciculi is indicated by a slight surface furrow, most evident in the upper (cranial or rostral) end of the spinal cord. The *fasciculus gracilis* is composed of fibres derived from the coccygeal, sacral, lumbar and lower thoracic spinal nerves arranged in that order from the midline outwards. The *fasciculus cuneatus* derives its fibres from the upper thoracic and cervical spinal nerves and is confined to the upper half of the spinal cord. The fibres in these fasciculi end in the *nucleus gracilis* and *nucleus cuneatus* respectively in the lower part of the medulla oblongata, where they synapse with the *secondary sensory neurons*. The axons from the latter cells, called collectively the *internal arcuate fibres*, pass ventromedially and cross the midline forming the great *medullary sensory decussation* (Fig. 19). Other fibres which have ascended in the lateral part of the fasciculus cuneatus are concerned with unconscious proprioception and enter the cerebellum (see page 95).

After crossing the midline, the internal arcuate fibres turn upwards and run cranially through the brain stem as the *medial lemniscus* to reach the ventrolateral thalamic nuclei where they synapse with the *tertiary sensory neurons*. The axons from the latter neurons proceed through the posterior limb of the internal capsule to the sensory cortex (see above).

Spinothalamic – spinal lemniscal system
Dorsal root afferent fibres mediating pain and temperature, enter the dorsolateral fasciculus (zone of Lissauer). Here they give rise to ascending and descending branches which traverse one or two segments of the spinal cord before entering the dorsal horn of the grey matter and its substantia gelatinosa to synapse with *second order neurons*.

The afferent fibres mediating light touch and pressure, on entering the spinal cord divide into branches which ascend and descend in the lateral part of the dorsal white column for several segments. These give off collaterals which enter the grey matter of the spinal cord to synapse with *second order neurons* and with intermediate neurons for spinal cord reflexes. Thus fibres conveying the sensations of touch and pressure are spread over several segments of the spinal cord.

The axons from the *second order neurons* cross the midline of the spinal cord in the ventral part of the grey matter or in the white commissure and proceed to the opposite side of the cord where they turn and pass upwards (cranially or rostrally) in the ventral and lateral white columns as two rather diffuse pathways, the *ventral* and *lateral spinothalamic tracts* (Figs. 46 and 47). The ventral tract carries impulses mainly concerned with tactile and pressure sensations; the lateral tract conveys impulses mediating pain and temperature sensations.

When crossing the spinal cord, the fibres from the second order neurons going to form the lateral spinothalamic tract lie nearer to the central canal of the spinal cord and are therefore more likely to be involved in pathological conditions which produce dilation of the central canal.

In the medulla oblongata the two spinothalamic tracts become blended to form the *spinal lemniscus* which in turn becomes closely associated in the brain stem with corresponding fibres from the fifth cranial nerve (*the trigeminal lemniscus*).

The spinal, trigeminal and medial lemnisci (see above) lie adjacent to each other and are partially commingled in their course through the pons and midbrain. The fibres of these various tracts end by forming synapses with cells of the *third order sensory neurons* in the ventrolateral nucleus of the thalamus. The axons of these third order neurons pass through the posterior limb of the internal capsule and corona radiata to end in the postcentral gyrus.

An unknown proportion of fibres in all the lemniscal systems (medial, spinal and trigeminal) give off collaterals to reticular nuclei or actually end by forming synapses with neurons in the reticular formation. These fibres form part of the input into the so-called afferent or ascending reticular system. This system is apparently involved in the arousal reaction and in autonomic, e.g. vascular and visceral, responses to painful and other afferent stimuli. (For additional information refer back to the Reticular Formation pp. 41–43).

The cerebellar tracts

The cerebellum, like the cerebrum, possesses both afferent and efferent pathways which enter or leave the cerebellum through its peduncles. Afferent fibres conveying information from muscle spindles, Golgi tendon organs, and touch and pressure receptors concerned with unconscious proprioception reach the cerebellum by various routes. There are three main ascending cerebellar pathways in each half of the spinal cord – *dorsal* and *ventral spinocerebellar tracts* and a third group of fibres ascending in the homolateral cuneate fasciculus adjacent to the posterior column of spinal grey matter, which form synapses in the accessory cuneate nucleus before proceeding to the cerebellum as the *dorsal external arcuate (cuneocerebellar)* fibres.

Dorsal (posterior) spinocerebellar tract

Some of the fibres conveying proprioceptive impulses from the lower limb and lower part of the trunk form synapses around cells in the thoracic nuclei (Clarke's columns) situated near the bases of the dorsal horns of spinal grey matter. These nuclei are most evident in the lower cervical, thoracic and upper lumbar segments of the spinal cord. The large diameter, and therefore rapidly conducting, axons from the thoracic nuclear cells ascend in the *homolateral dorsal spinocerebellar tract* (Fig. 46) to enter the cerebellum through its caudal peduncle.

Ventral (anterior) spinocerebellar tract

Other fibres conveying proprioceptive impulses synapse with different cells in the dorsal horns of grey matter in the lumbar and sacral segments of the spinal cord. A fresh relay of fibres arising from these dorsal cornual cells ascend mainly in the *ventral spinocerebellar tract* of the *same* side, but some cross in the cord to run upwards in the corresponding *heterolateral* tract; both tracts ascend through the spinal cord and brain stem to the level of the midbrain where they bend backwards to enter the cerebellum through the cranial cerebellar peduncles.

Dorsal (posterior) external arcuate (cuneocerebellar) fibres
A proportion of the nerve fibres conveying proprioceptive information from the upper half of the body and upper limbs do not form synapses in the spinal cord. On entering the cord these fibres turn upwards in the homolateral cuneate fasciculus and end in the *accessory cuneate nucleus* situated lateral to the main cuneate nucleus in the dorsal part of the medulla oblongata. The cells of the accessory cuneate nuclei are homologous with those in the thoracic nuclei, and their axons reach the cerebellum through the homolateral caudal cerebellar peduncle as the *dorsal external arcuate (cuneocerebellar) fibres*.

Other afferent fibres from the olivary (olivocerebellar tracts) and vestibular (vestibulocerebellar tracts) nuclei reach the cerebellum through the caudal cerebellar peduncles, and some from the colliculi (tectocerebellar fibres) and red nucleus (rubrocerebellar fibres) reach it through the cranial cerebellar peduncles.

Further large and very important afferent pathways, the *corticoponticerebellar pathways*, enter the cerebellum through the *middle cerebellar peduncles*. The fibres of these pathways arise from cells in the *cerebral cortex*, chiefly in the frontal, parietal and temporal regions, and descend through the corona radiata, internal capsules and cerebral peduncles to form synapses with cells in the pontine nuclei. Fresh relays of fibres cross transversely through the pons and enter the *opposite* pontine (middle) cerebellar peduncle to reach the middle lobe of the cerebellum.

The various afferent fibres entering through the cerebellar peduncles climb up to form synapses with the large flask-shaped Purkinje and other cells in the cerebellar cortex.

Efferent fibres
Efferent fibres arise from the Purkinje cells in the cerebellar cortex and arborize around other cells in nuclei, such as the dentate nucleus, situated within the central white matter of the cerebellum. The axons from cells in these nuclei enter the cranial (superior) cerebellar peduncles and *cross* to the opposite side in the lower half of

the midbrain. They end mainly in the heterolateral red nucleus (cerebellorubral or dentatorubral tract) although a proportion proceed to the other mesencephalic nuclei or end in the ventrolateral nucleus of the thalamus. By a further relay of fibres from the latter nucleus cerebellar influences are projected to the cerebral cortex. Some efferents which leave via the cranial peduncles descend in the brain stem to end in reticular and other nuclei. Efferent fibres also leave via the caudal (inferior) peduncle and terminate in the vestibular and other brain stem nuclei.

THE AUTONOMIC NERVOUS SYSTEM

The nervous system is subdivided into somatic and autonomic components chiefly on functional grounds, but anatomically they are neither separate nor distinct. They originate from the same primordial cells, they develop together, they are built up from the same basic units (neurons), associated in similar reflex arcs, they comprise central and peripheral parts and structurally they are always related and often closely connected. Any separation therefore is artificial rather than fundamental.

The autonomic nervous system regulates all those bodily processes which are not under voluntary or volitional control, with the exception of activities such as postural tonus. It consists of central and peripheral parts. The former are intrinsic parts of the central nervous system, being located in the cerebral cortex, hypothalamus, cerebellum, brain stem and spinal cord, and they are interconnected by various tracts. The latter consist of two paravertebral ganglionated trunks; various prevertebral and visceral nerve plexuses (cardiac, pulmonary, coeliac and hypogastric) and their branches in the neck, thorax, abdomen and pelvis; and autonomic fibres which are inherent constituents of most cranial and spinal nerves.

The *autonomic component* is mainly concerned with the regulation of circulatory, respiratory, alimentary, excretory and other visceral functions, being closely associated in some of these activities with certain ductless glands such as the pituitary and suprarenals. To effect this control it receives stimuli from the heart, vessels, lungs, alimentary tract, kidneys and other viscera, and transmits appropriate impulses to the same structures.

The functional units in both autonomic and somatic subdivisions are constructed from the same structural units or neurons linked together in chains of varying complexity. Common types of autonomic and somatic reflex arcs are illustrated in Fig. 7 and their basic similarity will be apparent. In the somatic system the entire inter-

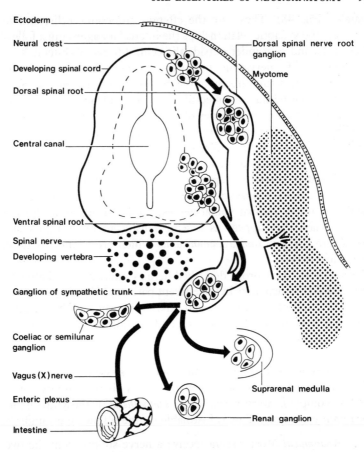

Fig. 48 Diagram showing the routes followed by cells migrating from the central nervous system along the spinal and vagus nerves. The former end up as dorsal nerve root ganglia, sympathetic trunk ganglia, as ganglia in prevertebral plexuses and as the cells of the suprarenal medulla. The latter are the main source of the nerve cells in the ganglia of the enteric plexuses, in intrinsic cardiac ganglia, etc.

calary (connector) neuron is within the central nervous system, whereas in the autonomic system the cell body of the intercalary neuron lies within the central nervous system but part of its axon travels outside, often for a considerable distance, to reach the ganglion in which the efferent cell bodies are situated. Fundamentally, therefore, there is no real difference in the arrangement, but merely a difference in the location of the cell bodies of the efferent neurons. Originally the autonomic and somatic components of the nervous system develop together, but at a later date in embryonic life groups of cells migrate outwards along the nerve roots to form peripheral ganglia (Fig. 48). These are the efferent autonomic cells, and to maintain the synaptic relationships the intercalary axons must follow these cells and so wander outside the central nervous system.

The mode of innervation of the suprarenal glands is unique as the intercalary fibres run directly to the medulla, with no synapse intervening. This is because the medulla is developed from migrant nerve cells which are the homologues of sympathetic efferent neurons.

The intercalary axons are termed *preganglionic* because they pass to the ganglia and the efferent fibres are termed *postganglionic* because they lie beyond the ganglia (Fig. 54). The former are myelinated and in mass they appear creamy white and constitute the *white rami communicantes* which are typically associated with the thoracic and upper lumbar spinal nerves; the latter are unmyelinated and in mass they appear as a semi-translucent greyish-pink and constitute the *grey rami communicantes* which are connected to all the spinal nerves.

Sometimes the neurons described here as intercalary and efferent are regarded as two links in the efferent pathway. It is simpler, however, to think of the afferent and efferent neurons as the terminal elements at each end of a reflex arc, and the link or links in between as intercalary or connector.

The subdivision of the autonomic nervous system

The autonomic part of the nervous system is divided into two more or less complementary parts — the *sympathetic* (orthosympathetic) and *parasympathetic*. This is justifiable on the following grounds:

1. *Anatomical* Most viscera receive a nerve supply from the two sources.
2. *Physiological* For most of these viscera the effects of the two nerve supplies are antagonistic.
3. *Pharmacological* Certain drugs which stimulate or inhibit sympathetic synapses or nerve terminals (endings) do not affect the parasympathetic and vice versa.

Mediation at the terminals of the parasympathetic postganglionic fibres is produced by acetylcholine as the neurotransmitter substance, so they are called cholinergic fibres. With some exceptions, e.g. sympathetic sudomotor fibres which are cholinergic, the postganglionic sympathetic fibre terminals utilise noradrenaline as their transmitter substance and are termed adrenergic (noradrenergic) fibres. Although mediation at synapses in autonomic ganglia is cholinergic, they are not all pharmacologically identical and indeed other chemical substances may sometimes be implicated.

In autonomic ganglia, especially sympathetic ganglia, the post-ganglionic fibres leaving outnumber the preganglionic fibres entering the ganglia. Thus the entering fibres must synapse with a larger number of efferent neurons giving off postganglionic fibres, thereby favouring more diffuse autonomic responses.

Highly specialised efferent nerve endings corresponding to motor end-plates in striated muscle cannot be demonstrated in the unstriated involuntary muscle of viscera and vessels, although specialised endings such as lamellated corpusles, which subserve afferent functions, may be found in or near these structures. Near, or within, the involuntary muscle to be innervated, adrenergic and cholinergic nerve fibres branch and intermingle to form an 'autonomic ground plexus'. Individual axons have a beaded appearance due to intermittent varicosities where they lose part of their neurolemmal (Schwann) cell coverings. These are the presumed sites of chemical transmitter release. Many of the cells in autonomic ground plexuses are neurolemmal (Schwann) or connective tissue cells. In some plexuses, such as the enteric, special neurons intervene between the terminations of the postganglionic efferent fibres and the structures innervated.

Only a small proportion of visceral and vascular unstriated muscle cells have transmitter-releasing axon varicosities on or near them; neighbouring cells are stimulated either by electrical activity from adjacent muscle cells or by diffusion of the chemical transmitter.

Although many of the terminal autonomic networks (ground plexuses) subserve efferent functions, similar arrangements of nerve fibres are also present in the depressor aortic area, the carotid sinus and various other reflexogenous zones which are known to be the sites of origin of important afferent stimuli. The exact nature of these terminal networks is a matter of controversy. Whatever their true nature, it is curious that they apparently occur only in areas where autonomic fibres terminate.

Autonomic representation in the central nervous system

The autonomic component, like the somatic, is controlled by higher 'centres' (groups of cells with related functions) in the central nervous system and the activities of all these 'centres' are closely integrated. It is well known that unpleasant sensations or strong emotions may cause visceral or vascular disturbances such as nausea, flushing or urinary frequency; these reactions provide evidence of the close connections existing between different parts of the brain. The integration of somatic and autonomic activities enables the body to maintain stable internal conditions despite changes in the envi-

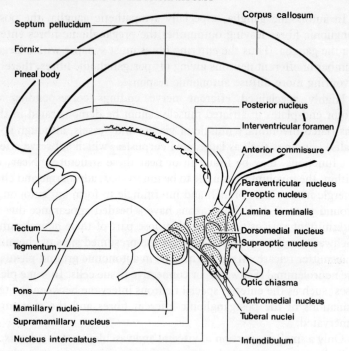

Fig. 49 The more important hypothalamic nuclei.

ronment, and ensures that circulatory, respiratory and other vital processes are controlled in accordance with general and local requirements. There is representation at cerebral cortical level in the frontal lobes and in the cingulate gyri; in the hippocampus; in the anterior lobe of the cerebellum; and in the hypothalamus, brain stem and spinal cord.

The hypothalamus is of especial autonomic importance and various nuclei have been distinguished in the hypothalamic parts of the lateral wall and floor of the third ventricle. Of these the most important are: (1) supraoptic, (2) paraventricular, (3) dorsal and ventral medial hypothalamic, (4) posterior hypothalamic and (5) mamillary (Fig. 49).

The hypothalamus has two-way interconnections with parts of the frontal lobes (Figs. 32 and 33). The supraoptic and paraventricular neclei have close interconnections with the posterior lobe of the pituitary gland (neurohypophysis) through the supraoptico-hypophysial tract. Furthermore the supraoptic nuclei may be concerned with parasympathetic activities, the paraventricular with sympathetic activities, and other nuclei with both.

Fibres from each hippocampus pass through the fornix to the homolateral medial mamillary nucleus where they relay. The axons of these mamillary neurons proceed through the mamillothalamic fasciculus to the homolateral anterior thalamic nucleus where they relay. The axons if these thalamic neurons project mainly to the cingulate gyrus, which is connected by association fibres in the cingulum to the hippocampus. This is the so-called 'hippocampal circuit' (hippocampus → fornix → mamillary body → anterior thalamic nucleus → cingulate gyrus → cingulum → hippocampus) which apparently maintains a continuous cycle of functional relationship between the cortex, thalamus, hypothalamus and hippocampal formation (p. 67). It is not a closed circuit, as it is influenced by hypothalamic ascending pathways from the spinal cord and brain stem and by descending corticohypothalamic pathways, and it and the associated parts of the brain correspond more or less closely to what has been referred to by various writers as the *limbic lobe or system*, the *autonomic brain*, or some other inadequate terms; for example 'autonomic brain' is an oversimplification, because other parts of the brain are also involved in autonomic activities. There is evidence, however, that the structrues implicated in the 'hippocampal circuit' are involved in emotional reactions, which are often the result of autonomic and somatic interactions, and perhaps with some forms of memory, and so it has attracted considerable physiological and psychiatric interest.

The hypothalamus is certainly involved in the control of visceral, cardiovascular and emotional responses; in regulating body-temperature, the sleep-waking rhythm and the endocrine system; and in maintaining constancy in the internal conditions by exercising control over the delicate yet precise adjustments to bodily environment.

In the brain stem the autonomic 'centres' are closely related to, or form parts of, the nuclei of origin of the third, seventh, ninth, tenth and eleventh cranial nerves.

In the spinal cord the autonomic cells giving off the preganglionic fibres are mainly located in the lateral grey columns, while the cell bodies of the secondary neurons of the afferent pathways lie mainly in the dorsal grey columns. The primary autonomic sensory neurons, like those of the somatic components, are located in dorsal spinal root ganglia and in ganglia associated with certain cranial nerves (Figs. 50 and 51).

The pathways connecting the various 'centres' in the hypothalamus brain stem and cord are not exactly known, but there is evidence that the main descending pathways run through the

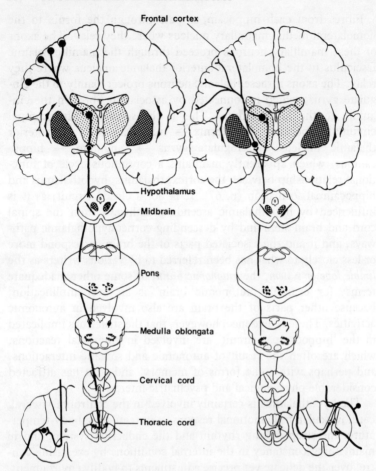

Fig. 50 Diagram showing probable routes of descending (efferent) autonomic pathways from the brain to the cord.

Fig. 51 Diagram showing probable routes of ascending (afferent) autonomic pathways from the cord to the brain.

dorsalateral parts of the tegmentum of the midbrain and pons, through the lateral parts of the reticular formation in the medulla oblongata and then in the ventral and lateral regions of the spinal cord (Fig. 50). Most of the fibres remain homolateral but others decussate both in the brain stem and cord.

Autonomic afferent fibres ascend through the cord and brain stem alongside the somatic sensory pathways, but whereas the majority of the fibres in the latter proceed to the thalamus, many of the autonomic afferent fibres probably run to the hypothalamus (Fig. 51).

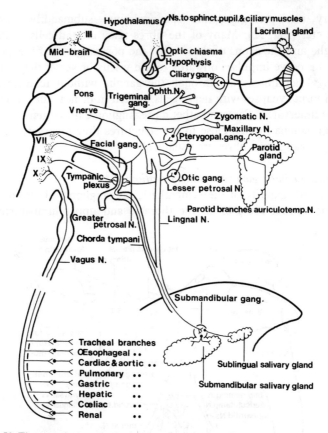

Fig. 52 The more important cranial parasympathetic pathways.

The hypothalamus may act as a relaying and redistributing centre from which the impulses are projected onwards to the thalamus and frontal cortex.

Autonomic outflows
Preganglionic fibres emerge from the central nervous system mainly from three regions:

The brain stem (cranial outflow)
The fibres are *parasympathetic* and form constituent parts of the third, seventh, ninth, tenth and eleventh cranial nerves. They run with these nerves for variable distances and leave them as fine branches (some named, e.g. chorda tympani, petrosal nerves, cardiac nerves, but most unnamed)which pass to ganglia such as the

ciliary, otic, pterygopalatine (spenopalatine), submandibular, cardiac etc. (Fig. 52). Many of the fibres relay around cells in these ganglia and the axons of these cells, the postganglionic fibres, convey the nerve impulses onwards to the viscus or vessel they innervate. Other fibres pass through the ganglia without relaying and then form synapses with nerve cells located in or near the structure to be innervated. Parasympathetic preganglionic fibres generally relay in ganglia located close to the structures they innervate and so the postganglionic fibres are usually short.

Thoracolumbar region (sympathetic outflow)
The great majority of the sympathetic preganglionic fibres emerge in the ventral roots of all the thoracic and upper lumbar spinal

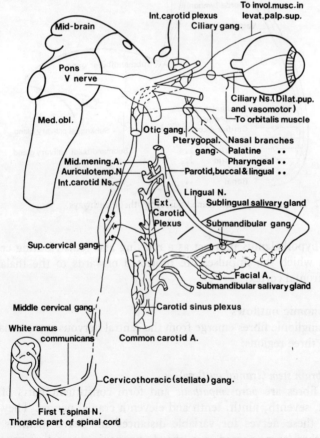

Fig. 53 The more important sympathetic pathways to various structures in the head.

nerves. They are the axons of cells located in the lateral grey columns of the cord. The fibres leave the spinal nerves as *white rami communicantes* which pass to adjacent ganglia in the paravertebral sympathetic trunks. Some relay in an adjacent ganglion; others pass upwards or downwards in the trunks before relaying in higher or lower ganglia, e.g. the fibres carrying impulses for the head end of the body emerge in the upper thoracic spinal nerves and run upwards to relay in the cervical ganglia of the sympathetic trunks (Fig. 53) and those for the lower limbs emerge in the lowest thoracic and upper lumbar spinal nerves and relay in the lumbar and sacral ganglia of the sympathetic trunks; and still others run through these trunks, without relaying, and pass in medially directed branches from these trunks, such as the cardiac and thoracic and lumbar splanchnic nerves, to the cardiac, coeliac and other autonomic plexuses where they end by forming synapses with efferent cells.

The axons of the ganglionic cells, the postganglionic fibres, may therefore be of considerable length, e.g. fibres supplying the vessels and sweat glands in the feet. Others, e.g. those passing to viscera and vessels within the thorax and abdomen, may be relatively short.

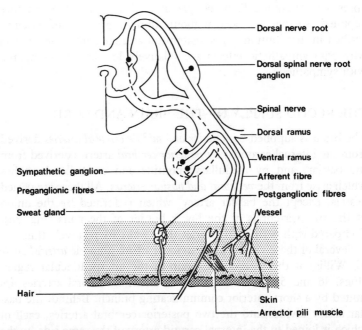

Fig. 54 This diagram shows how sympathetic postganglionic fibres accompany spinal nerves and supply, such structures as sweat glands, blood vessels and arrectores pilorum muscles.

The postganglionic fibres supplying structures in the head and neck, parietes and extremities usually join the relevant cranial and spinal nerves and are distributed with them. They are found in the *grey rami communicantes* interconnecting the ganglia of the paravertebral sympathetic trunks with nearby nerves. Each spinal nerve receives one or more grey rami and the constituent postganglionic fibres are distributed with these nerves and their branches to vessels, sweat glands, arrectores pilorum, etc., in their territories of distribution (Fig. 54).

The sacral outflow

Like the cranial outflow this is parasympathetic, and the fibres emerge in the second, third and fourth sacral nerves. They leave these nerves as a variable number of filaments, the *pelvic splanchnic nerves* (nervi erigentes), which pass directly to the inferior hypogastric (pelvic) plexuses. Some fibres relay in the ganglia within these plexuses and others pass through them to form synapses around cells in microscopic ganglia situated in or near the viscus or vessels they innervate. Thus the arrangement conforms to that of the cranial parasympathetic outflow – long preganglionic fibres forming synapses with efferent cells in ganglia situated near or in the structure supplied, so that the postganglionic fibres are short and circumscribed in distribution. This anatomical arrangement is one reason why parasympathetic effects are relatively localized as compared with sympathetic.

THE BLOOD SUPPLY OF THE BRAIN AND CORD

The brain is supplied by *anterior and middle cerebral arteries* derived from the internal carotids; by *posterior cerebral* arteries derived from the basilar, and by medullary, pontine and cerebellar branches which arise from the *vertebral and basilar arteries*. All these are paried vessels, except the basilar artery, which is formed by the union of the two vertebrals at the lower border of the pons (Fig. 36). Compared with peripheral arteries their walls are relatively thin.

Several of these vessels unite to form an anastomotic *arterial circle* (of Willis) at the base of the brain in the interpeduncular region (Figs. 36 and 55). In front the two anterior cerebral arteries are united by a short anterior communicating branch. Behind, the basilar artery divides into the two posterior cerebral arteries, each of which is joined to the internal carotid artery of the same side by the posterior communicating artery, and this vessel lies almost opposite the origin of the anterior cerebral artery.

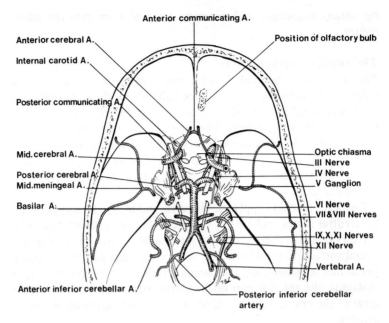

Fig. 55 The base of the cranium viewed from above, showing the cerebral arterial circle (of Willis) and the points of exit of the cranial nerves from skull.

The cerebral arteries give rise to *central* and *cortical* branches which do not anastomose with one another. The former supply the thalami, the corpus striatum, and adjacent parts of the brain such as the internal capsule, whereas the latter ramify in the pia mater and supply the cortex and subjacent areas. Due to the inadequate anastomoses between them a zone of diminished nutrition may exist between the areas supplied by the central and cortical vessels.

The *central vessels* are all derived from the arterial circle, or vessels close to it, and form six principal groups – anteromedial, postero-medial, right and left anterolateral and right and left posterolateral. They are 'end' arteries: that is they proceed to their terminations without forming any anastomoses with neighbouring vessels except through capillaries, and if one is blocked for any reason the area of brain supplied by it degenerates.

The *cortical vessels* are the terminal branches of the anterior, middle and posterior cerebral arteries and they ramify in the pia mater, anastomosing at this level. They give off branches which penetrate the brain substance perpendicularly and these do not anastomose, or only communicate through delicate vessels, so that in effect they resemble 'end' arteries. Some are very short and end in the cortex, but others are longer and penetrate for 2 to 6 cm into the white matter.

The anterior cerebral artery

This arises near the medial end of the stem of the lateral cerebral sulcus and passes forwards and medially above the optic nerve to the longitudinal fissure, where it is united to its fellow by the anterior communicating artery. The two arteries thereafter run close together in the longitudinal fissure, following the curve of the corpus callosum upon which they rest. In the region of the splenium and precuneus they end by anastomosing with branches of the posterior cerebral arteries.

Cortical branches supply the cingulate and medial frontal gyri, the paracentral lobule and part of the precuneus, in addition to a strip corresponding to these areas along the adjacent part of the superolateral surface. Central branches pierce the medial part of the rostral perforated substance and the lamina terminalis to supply the hypothalamus, the anterior part of the corpus striatum and the adjacent areas of the brain; these constitute the *anteromedial* group of central arteries.

The middle cerebral artery

This is the largest branch of the internal carotid artery and its direct continuation. It runs outwards to the insula in the stem of the lateral sulcus and divides into cortical branches which supply the orbital surfaces and the insula and most of the superolateral surface of the brain, except fringes round the borders which are supplied by the anterior and posterior cerebral arteries.

Near its origin it gives off an *anterolateral* (thalamostriate) group of central branches which penetrate the lateral part of the rostral perforated substance to supply the caudate and lentiform nuclei, much of the internal capsule and part of the thalamus; rupture of one of these vessels and the resulting haemorrhage is the commonest cause of cerebral apoplexy ('shock' or 'stroke').

The posterior cerebral arteries

These are the two terminal branches of the basilar artery. Passing outwards, each receives the posterior communicating branch from the corresponding internal carotid artery, and then winds backwards between the cerebral peduncle and uncus to reach the tentorial surface of the cerebrum where it divides into branches for the supply of the temporal and occipital lobes. They supply the parahippocampal, lingual, and medial and lateral occipitotemporal gyri and also the cuneus, part of the precuneus and the outer surface of the occipital lobe.

They give off a group of *posteromedial* central branches which enter the brain through the interpeduncular perforated substance and help to supply the thalamus, lentiform nucleus, internal capsule and lateral wall of the third ventricle. They also supply a group of *posterolateral* central branches which penetrate and supply the cerebral peduncles, the pulvinar of the thalamus, the tectum of the mid-brain and the pineal and geniculate bodies.

Small *posterior choroidal arteries*, usually 3 to 5 in number, arise from the posterior cerebral arteries opposite the cerebral peduncles. The more anterior vessels cross the geniculate bodies, help to supply them, and then enter the choroidal plexuses in the posterior part of the temporal horn of the lateral ventricle through the lower part of the choroidal fissure. The others curve around the pulvinar to enter the tela choroidea and supply branches to parts of the choroid plexuses of the lateral and third ventricles, to the fornix, to the thalamus and to the midbrain.

The *anterior choroidal arteries*, usually one on each side, arise from the internal carotids between the origins of the posterior communicating and middle cerebral arteries. Passing backwards and inwards across the corresponding optic tract, each then lies along the medial side of the tract until it reaches the lateral geniculate body. Here it splits up into branches, most of which turn outwards and recross the optic tract to enter the corresponding temporal horn of the lateral ventricle through the choroidal fissure where they supply the choroid plexus in that region. These choroidal arteries also supply twigs to the optic tracts, hypothalamus, midbrain and lateral geniculate bodies, and others penetrate the cerebrum to supply the posterior limb of the internal capsule, the optic radiations and adjacent parts of the corpus striatum and rhinencephalon.

The part played by the choroidal arteries in supplying various parts of the optic pathways and geniculate bodies is noteworthy.

The basilar artery

This supplies pontine, anterior inferior cerebellar, labyrinthine and superior cerebellar branches, in addition to the larger posterior cerebral arteries. They supply the pons, the anteroinferior and superior parts of the cerebellum, and the internal ear.

The vertebral arteries

These give off anterior and posterior spinal, posterior inferior cerebellar, choroidal, meningeal and medullary branches.

The two *anterior spinal* arteries unite to form a single median vessel which runs downwards on the cord. The corresponding *posterior* spinal arteries descend along the lines of the posterior nerve roots. All are reinforced by spinal branches of other arteries.

The posterior inferior *cerebellar* branch supplies the corresponding aspects of the cerebellum, and the *choroid* vessels end in the choroid plexus of the fourth ventricle.

The branches supplying the nuclei and tracts in the medulla, like the central arteries described above, are insignificant in size, but are nevertheless very important because of the cardiac, respiratory and other 'vital' centres within their territories of supply.

The spinal cord
As they descend the anterior and posterior spinal arteries are reinforced by a series of small spinal arteries which arise from the vertebral, ascending cervical, posterior intercostal and lumbar arteries. These are united by longitudinal branches which lie in the midline anteriorly and close to the lines of emergence of the posterior nerve roots. The reinforcing arteries vary in size and are usually largest in the lower cervical and thoracolumbar regions opposite the cervical and lumbar enlargements (Fig. 9). They enter the spinal canal through the intervertebral foramina.

The veins of the brain
These have very thin walls and no valves and they end in the venous sinuses of the dura mater. They may be divided into external or cortical and internal or central groups.

There are three main groups of external cerebral veins on each side – superior, middle and inferior.

The *superior cerebral veins* ascend obliquely over the superolateral and medial surfaces of the hemispheres and drain into the superior sagittal sinus.

There are *superficial and deep middle cerebral veins* and they lie in the lateral sulcus. They are formed by the union of several smaller cortical veins and tributaries from adjacent subcortical areas. The superficial vein drains into the cavernous sinus and communicates directly through *superior and inferior anastomotic veins* with the superior sagittal and transverse sinuses respectively. The deep vein lies in the depths of the lateral sulcus and unites with the anterior cerebral, insular, inferior thalamostriate, inferior choroidal and anterolateral (thalamostriate) veins to form the basal vein. The right and left basal veins are formed near the rostral perforated substance. Each runs backwards around the cerebral peduncle to end in the great cerebral vein. In addition to the tributaries already mentioned, it receives others from structures in the interpeduncular fossa, the temporal horn of the lateral ventricle, the parahippocampal gyrus and the midbrain.

Numerous *inferior cerebral veins* drain the inferior surfaces of the hemispheres and open into adjacent venous sinuses or the basal vein.

The *internal cerebral veins* drain the deeper parts of the hemispheres and ultimately form two main channels by the union of the superior thalamostriate and superior choroidal veins near the interventricular foramina. These internal cerebral veins run backwards close to the midline, between the layers of the tela choroidea, and unite beneath the splenium to form the *great cerebral vein* (Galen) which is joined by the basal veins before entering the commencement of the straight sinus.

The cerebellar veins end in the straight, transverse, sigmoid and petrosal sinuses.

The veins of the cord drain into the internal vertebral venous plexuses and they in turn drain into the extensive external vertebral venous plexuses, which end in the vertebral, azygos, hemiazygos and lumbar veins.

THE DEVELOPMENT OF THE NERVOUS SYSTEM

The nervous system originates from a dorsal midline ectodermal thickening termed the *neural plate*, which soon becomes infolded to form first a *neural groove* and later a *neural tube* (Figs. 56 and 57). The unclosed ends remain patent for a short time and form communications (cranial and caudal neuropores) with the amniotic cavity: these are closed by the end of the fourth week. The region of the cranial neuropore is probably represented later by the lamina terminalis. The neural tube becomes separated from the surface ectoderm by the interposition of mesoderm cells and it lies immediately dorsal to the notochord. For a time its caudal part is in communication with the hindgut by a small opening, the neurenteric canal, which represents the persisting original blastopore and notochordal canal. The walls of the neural tube become thickened by cellular proliferation and at the head end it becomes expanded irregularly to form *fore-, mid- and hindbrain vesicles* from which the brain is derived. The remainder of the neural tube retains its pristine shape and becomes the spinal cord. This stage in the development of the central nervous system is reached by the end of the fifth week

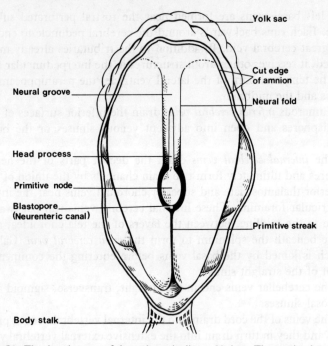

Fig. 56   The dorsal aspect of the embryonic disc at 20 days. The amnion has been removed.

of intrauterine life. The development of the spinal cord will first be considered.

The spinal cord

The cord is developed from the caudal end of the neural tube. Before they close to form the neural tube, the margins of the neural groove become thickened and constitute the *neural crests*, which form a specialised column of cells on each side of the tube (Fig. 57). The peripheral parts of the somatic and autonomic nervous systems are derived from the neural tube, neural crests and to a minor extent at the head end from localised ectodermal thickenings or *placodes*. The cells in the neural crests proliferate opposite the somites, but not between, and so groups of neuroblasts are formed that later become the ganglia on the cranial and spinal nerves (Fig. 48).

Neuroblasts (the forerunners of definitive neurons) also migrate outwards from the neural tube and crests along the developing nerve roots for varying distances. Some become arrested at points alongside the primitive vertebrae and later form the ganglia of the sympathetic trunks, but others progress further, still retaining their

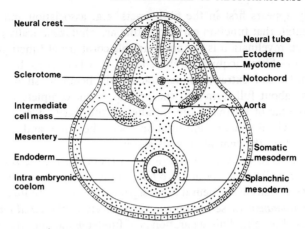

Fig. 57 Cross-section through a human embryo about 4 weeks old showing the neural tube and neural crests.

central connections, and ultimately constitute the ganglion cells in the prevertebral and visceral autonomic plexuses (Fig. 48). Incidentally the medullae of the suprarenals and the paraganglia (chromaffin cells) also arise from similar migrating neuroblasts.

The ectodermal neural tube becomes differentiated as a special neuroectoderm from which neuroblasts, spongioblasts and ependyma are derived. The neuroblasts give rise to neurons and the spongioblasts to neuroglia. By cellular proliferation the neural tube increases in length and thickness, although it lags behind the growth of its surroundings, and so it becomes progressively shorter than the vertebral column; in consequence the original segmental correspondence between nervous and vertebral elements is lost.

At first the central canal is oval, the walls consisting only of two or three layers of cells, but soon the lateral walls thicken and the lumen steadily narrows. The dorsal and ventral parts of the tube remain thin at this stage and are termed the roof and floor plates, and three zones, an inner *ependymal*, an intermediate *mantle* and an outer *marginal*, become definable. The first gives rise to ependymal cells and to others which migrate into the mantle layer. The mantle zone consists of neuroblasts and spongioblasts which later form the grey matter of the cord; and the marginal layer mainly forms a framework for the processes growing out from the neuroblasts in the mantle zone, i.e. for the future white matter. Some of the processes form intersegmental, association and commissural fibres and others become projection or itinerant fibres linking the brain and cord.

Myelination of the fibres commences about the fourth month and usually appears first in the fibre tracts. e.g. association and inter-segmental, that function earliest or that are phylogenetically oldest, although myelination is not an invariable corollary of function. The projection fibres acquire myelin sheaths at a later period, e.g. the pyramidal and extrapyramidal tracts only begin to show myelin sheaths about full term and the process is not complete until the second year of postnatal life. Studies of the times of myelination have provided valuable information about the origin and course of tracts within the central nervous system.

The cells in the ventral and dorsal parts of the mantle zone pro-liferate rapidly and produce two longitudinal bulges on each side in the lateral walls of the neural tube, separated by a longitudinal sulcus (*sulcus limitans*); these are known respectively as the *basal and alar laminae* (Fig. 58). This separation is of fundamental importance, for these laminae are associated respectively with efferent and afferent functions. The nerve cells in the basal lamina form the anterior and lateral grey columns which become associated with somatic (vol-untary) and autonomic (visceral) motor activities respectively, while those in the alar laminae mainly form secondary sensory neurons in afferent pathways: the autonomic columns lie adjacent to the sulcus limitans and the somatic columns nearer the roof and floor plates. Some basal neuroblasts send out processes through the mantle layer which become aggregated together into rootlets at the surface of the developing hindbrain and cord. These are the motor or ventral roots of the cranial and spinal nerves respectively. Coincident with this, pseudounipolar cells in the dorsal spinal and cranial nerve ganglia originating from the neural crests send out axons which divide in a

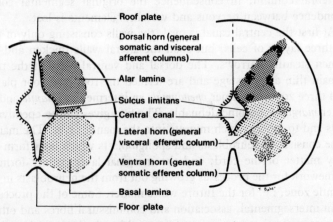

Fig. 58 A diagram showing the alar and basal laminae in the embryonic spinal cord and the columns of cells developed in them.

T-shaped fashion into central and peripheral processes; the former enter the neuraxis and constitute the sensory or afferent roots of the cranial and spinal nerves, and the latter extend outwards in these same nerves to special sensory endings in somatic or visceral structures. Efferent and afferent fibres are distinguishable as early as the fifth week of embryonic life.

The brain

The brain is developed from the enlargement and elaboration of the fore-, mid- and hindbrain vesicles (prosencephalon, mesencephalon and rhombencephalon) which are demarcated from each other and from the cord by shallow constrictions. The narrowing between the mid- and hindbrains is more definite than the others and is termed the isthmus rhombencephali.

At an early stage three flexures appear – cephalic, pontine and cervical.

When the head fold is formed the brain also is flexed forward in the region of the midbrain and this is known as the *cephalic or mesencephalic flexure* (Figs. 59 and 60). The forebrain becomes bent ventrally around the cranial extremity of the notochord and for a

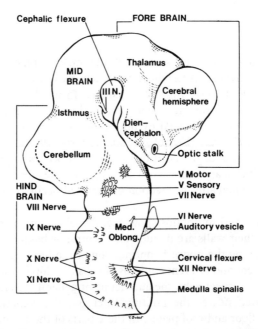

Fig. 59 Brain of human embryo about the 10 to 11 mm stage (modified from a model by His).

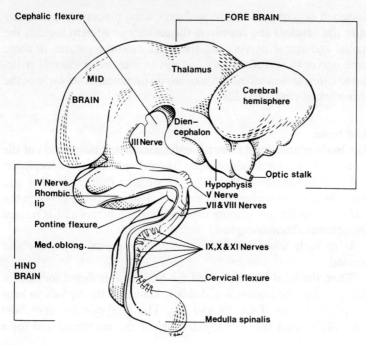

Fig. 60 Brain of human embryo about the 13 to 14 mm stage (modified from a model by His).

time the dorsal convex surface of the mesencephalon, opposite the cephalic flexure, is the most prominent part of the brain.

The *pontine flexure* (Fig. 60) is convex forwards, occurs in the future pontine region and is not associated with bending or folding of the head but is produced by unequal growth in the hindbrain.

The *cervical flexure* (Fig. 60) is concave forwards and is associated with the bending of the head on the neck. It occurs at the junction of the hindbrain and spinal cord and approximates to 90° at the seventh week. Thereafter as erection of the head occurs it is gradually abolished.

The hind- and midbrains show ependymal, mantle and marginal zones and their walls are divided into ventral or basal and dorsal or alar laminae by the upward continuation of the limiting sulci of the cord. Efferent and afferent columns of cells develop in the basal and alar laminae respectively, the autonomic or general visceral columns being located nearer the limiting sulci and the somatic columns nearer the floor and roof plates. In these parts of the brain, however, additional intermediate columns of cells develop between the efferent somatic and autonomic columns and also between the corre-

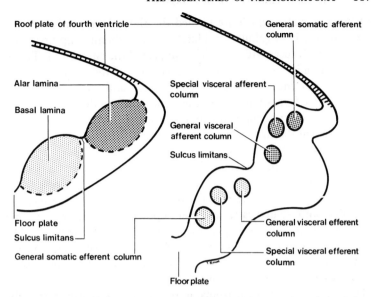

Fig. 61 A diagram showing the alar and basal laminae in the embryonic medulla oblongata and the columns of cells developed in them.

sponding afferent columns of cells. These are the special visceral (branchial) columns of cells (Fig. 61) and they innervate ultimately structures derived from the branchial arches. All these columns become interrupted to form the nuclei of various cranial nerves: for example, the somatic efferent column is represented by the third, fourth, sixth and twelfth nerve nuclei; the special visceral efferent column gives origin to the motor nuclei of the fifth and seventh nerves and the nucleus ambiguus of the tenth nerves; the general visceral efferent column (corresponding to the lateral grey column of the cord) forms the salivary nuclei of the seventh and ninth nerves and the dorsal nucleus of the tenth nerves, and so on.

The hindbrain (rhombencephalon)
This part of the brain increases both in length and width and the maximum width is opposite the pontine flexure. The widening is accompanied by a certain amount of flattening, the lateral walls falling outwards like the pages of an opening book, so that the alar laminae come to lie lateral rather than dorsal to the basal laminae. In consequence the roof plate also becomes stretched and widened and the cavity becomes somewhat rhomboidal in shape and subsequently forms the fourth ventricle.

The thin expanded roof plate is attached to the dorsilateral edges of the alar plates which are termed the rhombic lips (Fig. 60). As a result largely of cellular proliferation, each rhombic lip first overlaps and then fuses with the subjacent part of the lateral wall. Thereafter cells migrate from it into the vicinity of the basal lamina to form the pontine, olivary and arcuate nuclei and the grey matter of the reticular formation. About the same time the thin floor plate is invaded by decussating and commissural fibres and becomes thickened to form the median raphe.

The part of the hindbrain caudal to the pontine flexure, *the myelencephalon*, become the medulla oblongata, and the part on the cranial side, *the metencephalon*, gives rise to the pons and cerebellum.

The lower part of the medulla oblongata resembles the medulla spinalis both structurally and developmentally. The gracile and cuneate nuclei are developed from cells in the alar laminae. The upper part bounds the lower half of the fourth ventricle and the redisposition of the lateral walls, the thickening of the floor plate and the stretching and thinning of the roof plate have been described above. Descending corticospinal fibres invade the ventral part of the medulla oblongata about the fourth month and form the pyramids, and the afferent fibres ascending from the cord pass through the marginal zone adjacent to the alar laminae on their way to the cerebrum and cerebellum.

The metencephalon forms the pons and the cerebellum, the latter being developed from symmetrical thickenings of its alar plates and their rhombic lips. Its cavity constitutes the upper half of the fourth ventricle.

The arrangements of cell zones and columns is the same in the developing pons as in the medulla, and the nuclei of the fifth, sixth and seventh cranial nerves originate in them. About the fourth month corticospinal and corticopontine fibres penetrate between the pontine nuclei and so create the pontine bulge.

Initially the cerebellar anlagen (an anlage is the embryonic area in which traces of any part first appear, or the first aggregation of cells which will form any distinct part of an embryo) project as small, symmetrical bulges on the roof of the fourth ventricle. Later these increase in size and the central part of the roof plate is invaded by cells and forms the vermis interconnecting the two enlarging cerebellar hemispheres. In the earlier stages the cerebellum is stretched across the upper part of the fourth ventricle. Above it blends with the superior medullary velum, which is developed from the roof of the isthmus rhombencephali, and below with the tenuous roof plate of the myelencephalon.

The midbrain (mesencephalon)

This part of the brain undergoes least change during development. The same basic arrangement into zones and columns of cells occurs in the midbrain as in the cord and hindbrain. The third nerve nuclei and the grey matter of the reticular formation develop from cells in the basal laminae. The fourth nerve nuclei and the mesencephalic nuclei of the fifth nerves are formed in the junctional area, the isthmus rhombencephali between the mid- and hindbrains, and this part later becomes largely incorporated in the midbrain. The red nuclei and substantia nigra are probably derived from the cells of the basal laminae.

The colliculi originate from the alar laminae. The cells proliferate and invade the roof plate and the resulting thickened area is first subdivided by a vertical median groove and then subdivided again by a transverse furrow, In this way the tectum and colliculi are formed.

The cavity within the mesencephalon remains very narrow and forms the mesencephalic aqueduct which interconnects the third and fourth ventricles. Thickening of the wall is brought about by proliferation of the cells in both laminae and by the passage of itinerant fibres, such as the pyramidal and lemniscal tracts, which are superadded to existing structures.

The forebrain (prosencephalon)

To begin with the forebrain has thicker lateral walls, and thin roof and floor plates similar to those in other parts of the developing brain, and each lateral wall shows ventral and dorsal areas separated by a furrow which later becomes the hypothalamic sulcus.

During the fifth week the original forebrain vesicle develops bilateral outgrowths which expand rapidly to form the cerebral hemispheres (Fig. 62). These outgrowths from the original vesicle are termed the *telencephalon* and the remainder of the fore-brain vesicle is referred to as the *diencephalon*. At a still earlier stage, before the closure of the cranial neuropore, paired diverticula grow forwards from the forebrain: these are the optic vesicles and their distal parts expand and invaginate to form the retinae, from which nerve fibres grow backwards through the hollow optic stalks and convert them into the solid optic nerves. The cavities of the optic stalks and vesicles are obliterated, but those within the telecephalic vesicles form the lateral ventricles, and the unpaired central cavity within the diencephalon becomes the third ventricle; the openings between them persist as the interventricular foramina. The anterior part of

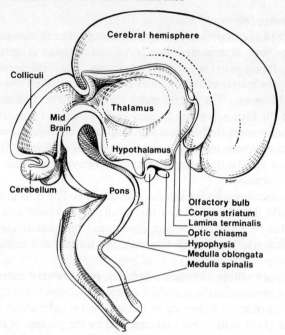

Fig. 62   Brain of human embryo about 3 months old (modified from a model by His).

the roof plate of the forebrain remains thin and forms the definitive lamina terminalis. Other paired diverticula from the floors of the telencephalic vesicles form the olfactory bulbs and tracts. These developments become evident during the second month.

The **diencephalon** gives rise to the thalami, geniculate and pineal bodies, the greater part of the hypothalamus, the roof of the third ventricle and the neurohypophysis (posterior lobe of the pituitary). The cavity is narrowed by the growth of the thalami in the alar plate of the diencephalon and ultimately forms a narrow cleft which is bridged by the interthalamic adhesion (connexus).

A groove at first separates each thalamus from the parts of the homolateral cerebral hemisphere which grows backwards. With increasing growth this disappears and the thalamus then comes into contact with the corpus striatum, but still later the developing itinerant or projection fibres passing to and from the cerebral cortex extend between them to form the internal capsule.

The geniculate bodies and habenula are initially in close relationship, but they are separated by the backward growth of the thalamus, a process that also excludes the geniculate bodies from their original position in the lateral walls of the third ventricle.

The caudal part of the roof plate is associated with the development of the pineal body and the fornical and posterior commissures. The anterior part remains thin and is invaginated by a rich plexus of vessels to form the choroid plexus of the third ventricle.

The floor plate forms part of the hypothalamus, including the tuber cinereum, the infundibulum, the posterior lobe of the hypophysis and the corpora mamillaria. The optic vesicles arise, before the separation into telencephalon and diencephalon is evident, from the part that subsequently becomes the diencephalon. The optic chiasma is regarded as the boundary between the subdivisions of the forebrain vesicles. The anterosuperior parts of the adult third ventricles are derived from the telencephalon.

The **telencephalon** thus consists of a median part and two lateral diverticula. The median portion is bounded anteroinferiorly by the lamina terminalis and forms part of the third ventricle and lateral wall of the hypothalamus.

The lateral diverticula outgrow and finally overlap all the other parts of the brain. They form ovoid hemispheres separated by a median longitudinal cleft or fissure. The walls are thin at first, but soon the neuroblasts in their mantle zones multiply profusely and some migrate peripherally to form the cerebral cortex. The cortex is smooth until the third month. Then a depression, the lateral cerebral fossa, appears on the lateral surface and it is converted subsequently into the insula and lateral cerebral sulcus, although the process is not completed until after birth. About the same time, or somewhat earlier, a shallow parahippocampal sulcus appears, but the other sulci are not evident before the fourth month and they are not all visible until about the end of the seventh month.

The ventral end of each hemisphere becomes the frontal pole. As enlargement proceeds, however, the original dorsal pole grows downwards and forwards to form the temporal pole and the superjacent part extends backwards and becomes the occipital pole. The contained cavity is distorted and pulled out by these movements and this explains the irregular shape of the lateral ventricles.

Each corpus striatum is formed by active cellular proliferation in the floor and in the adjacent part of the lateral wall of the lateral cerebral vesicle. The posterior end of the corpus striatum lies close to the original dorsal end of the cerebral vesicle which later grows downwards and forwards to form the temporal lobe and pole. In consequence part of the corpus is also carried downwards and forwards and is continued from the floor of the central part of the lateral ventricle into the roof of the temporal horn; this part becomes attenuated and comma shaped – the caudate nucleus. The changing relationships of the thalamus and corpus striatum and the origin of the internal capsule have been described above.

The medial walls of the cerebral vesicles become thickened, except along a line on each side extending from the interventricular foramen backwards and downwards within the curving margin of the fornix. These thin areas are invaginated by pia mater and become the choroid plexuses of the lateral ventricles, which are continuous with the corresponding plexus of the third ventricle at the interventricular foramina.

The development of the commissures produces considerable alterations. Most of these fibres appear initially in the region of the lamina terminalis and some, such as those of the anterior commissure, maintain this position. Others, such as the fibres of the commissura fornicis, move backwards, and this is associated with the phenomenal growth of the cerebral hemispheres and the development of the very large corpus callosum. The fibres of the corpus callosum lie within the lamina terminalis near the interventricular foramina, but as their numbers increase enormously the corpus increases in size, extending forwards, upwards and then backwards far beyond its original confines. The fibres of the commissura fornicis are carried backwards with it to their definitive position beneath the splenium. As the corpus callosum extends backwards it overlaps the roof of the third ventricle and a transverse slit or fissure is thus formed between it and the fornix above and the roof of the third ventricle below. This is occupied by the tela choroidea – a double fold of pia mater trapped between the roof of the diencephalon and the backward enlargement of the cerebral hemispheres with their commissural fibres.

PRACTICAL NEUROANATOMY

The instruments required for brain dissection are simple – scalpel, forceps, fine-pointed scissors, probe and a brain-knife (a knife with a long blade); the last should be provided by the institution or laboratory. Blunt dissection with a scalpel handle is often the best macroscopic method for tracing larger fibre tracts, e.g. association and commissural, but special histological, histochemical, electron-microscopical, experimental and other techniques must be used to obtain more accurate and detailed information. A skull with a removable 'cap' and a low-power magnifying lens should always be available.

Identify the main parts of the brain – cerebrum, cerebellum, midbrain, pons and medulla oblongata – and note their relationships to the skull. Many other parts can be examined only after the brain has undergone further dissection.

The frontal, occipital and temporal poles and the borders of the cerebrum are easily recognised, and by separating the lips of the longitudinal fissure (p. 49) the corpus callosum (p. 53) can be seen in its depths. The relationships of the temporal lobe, cerebellum and sigmoid sinus (p. 26) to the mastoid and petrous parts of the temporal bone, of the middle meningeal vessels at the pterion and the stem of the lateral sulcus to the lesser wing of the sphenoid bone, and of the many important structures in the region of the cavernous sinuses (p. 26), all deserve careful study; this will necessitate revising information already learned while dissecting the head.

Note the olfactory bulbs, tracts and striae (p. 66), the rostral (anterior) perforated substance (p. 66), and the optic nerves, chiasma and tracts (p. 77). The internal carotid and middle cerebral arteries (p. 108) are lateral to the chiasma, and behind it from before backwards are the infundibulum, tuber cinereum, mamillary bodies and interpeduncular (posterior) perforated substance forming the floor of the third ventricle (p. 76) and part of the hypothalamus (p. 74). The vertebral and basilar arteries (p. 108) lie respectively on the ventral aspects of the medulla oblongata and pons.

Study any remnants of the dura mater (p. 21) such as the falx cerebri, tentorium cerebelli, etc., and any remaining portions of the associated venous sinuses (pp. 25 to 27). Now examine the arachnoid, with its cisterns and granulations (pp. 27 to 28), and inspect a skull 'cap' for the impressions these granulations produce; they are most easily seen near the groove for the superior sagittal sinus. A small piece of arachnoid should be cut off, placed under water, and examined with a magnifying lens to see its web-like structure. Most brains available for anatomical dissection, however, have been 'fixed' and preserved in formalin and they seldom reveal the spider-web appearance by this manoeuvre. Lecturers supervising brain dissections, however, are often able to provide 'unfixed' specimens of arachnoid obtained from recent post-mortem examinations; these specimens will normally show the delicate structure of the arachnoid.

Complete the study of the meninges by observing the pia pater (p. 28) which follows closely all the surface irregularities of the brain. Identify also the small cauliflower-like protrusions of the choroid plexus through the lateral apertures of the fourth ventricle (p. 47).

At this stage the twelve pairs of cranial nerves and their points of emergence or superficial origins from the brain should be identified. Their deep or nuclear attachments, as stated on p. 127, can seldom be discerned unless specially stained sections are available for study.

1st (olfactory)

These are 20 to 30 filaments attached to the undersides of the olfactory bulbs (p. 66), which reach them by traversing the cribiform ethmoidal plate. They convey impulses from the olfactory areas of the nasal mucous membrane.

2nd (optic)

Each nerve, carrying visual impulses from the retina, passes backwards from the eye through the optic canal to the optic chiasma (p. 77). The retinae are diencephalic outgrowths (p. 119), so these nerves are invested by dural and arachnoid sheaths and by a prolongation of the subarachnoid space as far as the eyeballs. Thus any rise in the pressure of the cerebrospinal fluid may compress the optic nerves and central retinal arteries, producing visual disturbances and characteristic retinal changes. The dural and arachnoid sheaths around other cranial nerves are relatively short and soon fuse with the epineurium.

3rd (oculomotor)

These nerves emerge from grooves on the medial sides of the cerebral peduncles (p. 39) and run forwards lateral to the posterior communicating arteries. They are most important motor nerves supplying the extrinsic (voluntary) and instrinsic (involuntary) eye muscles.

4th (trochlear)

These slender nerves arise from the tectum of the midbrain immediately below the caudal colliculi and curve ventrally around the cerebral peduncles; at this stage of the dissecton the latter parts alone are visible. They are the only cranial nerves emerging from the dorsal aspect of the brain stem.

5th (trigeminal)

These are the largest cranial nerves. They are composed of stout sensory and much thinner motor roots which are attached to the side of the pons (p. 36), about midway between its upper and lower borders and about 2.5 cm from the midline. The trigeminal ganglia (p. 24) will almost certainly *not* be present in the specimens available for dissection.

6th (abducent) These appear on each side through the groove between the pons and the medullary pyramids (p. 32). They pierce the dura mater lateral to the sphenoidal dorsum sellae as they bend forwards over the apices of the petrous parts of the temporal bones.

7th (facial) and 8th (vestibulocochlear)

These nerves share a common dural and arachnoid sheath as they emerge in the cerebellopontine angle, anteromedial to the cerebellar flocculi and near the openings of the lateral recesses of the fourth ventricle (p. 46). The facial nerve lies medial to the vestibulocochlear, with the nervous intermedius of the facial nerve interposed between them.

9th (glossopharyngeal) 10th (vagus) and cranial roots of the 11th (accessory)

These nerves issue as a series of fine rootlets from the posterolateral sulci of the medulla oblongata (p. 32) in line from above downwards. The ninth nerve has its own dural and arachnoid sheath, but the tenth and eleventh nerves share a common sheath. *The spinal roots of the accessory nerves* arise by a series of rootlets from the lateral sides of the upper 5 or 6 cervical segments of the spinal cord. They coalesce as they ascend posterior to the ligamentum denticulatum to enter the skull through the foramen magnum, where they join the cranial roots to form the accessory nerve.

12th (hypoglossal)

These nerves appear as a series of rootlets through the anterolateral sulci of the medulla oblongata (p. 32). They unite on each side to form two main bundles which pierce the dura mater separately before uniting to form the definitive hypoglossal nerves.

Unfortunately the fragile rootlets of the 9th to 12th nerves are often avulsed partially or completely during removal of the brain from the skull, so it may be difficult or impossible to find them in many dissecting room specimens. Most students, however, will have access to a museum where perfect brain specimens are displayed.

The arteries and veins of the brain should now be studied in more detail, using the descriptions on pages 106 to 111, because many of them will be cut or removed during the subsequent dissection procedures. The main parts of the vessels lie in the subarachnoid space, and the walls of both cerebral arteries and veins are relatively so thin, in comparison with those of their peripheral counterparts, that the arteries may be mistaken for veins and the veins regarded as arachnoid strands. They can be beautifully displayed by differential injections of various red and blue substances, but the techniques are specialised and time-consuming, so most of the really good specimens are found in museums. The groups of fine central arteries can be detected by pulling gently on the parent anterior, middle and posterior cerebral arteries, while using a hand lens to magnify these delicate vessels.

The cerebral veins drain into the dural venous sinuses (pp. 25 to 27) and most of the blood ultimately enters the internal jugular veins; these sinuses and veins should have been studied previously during dissection of the head and neck. The sinuses communicate through emissary veins with veins of the scalp, face and neck, and receive most of the blood from the diploic veins. The shadows cast by diploic veins should be studied in radiographs of the skull, as they can be mistaken for fractures, especially those cast by the parietal group which are referred to rather fancifully as the 'parietal spider'.

The dura mater is supplied by meningeal arteries (p. 24) and their accompanying veins which lie between the arteries and the bone. Note the grooves in the skull produced by these vessels.

The brain stem and cerebellum
Holding the brain so that the frontal poles are inferior, gently separate the superior surface of the cerebellum from the tentorial surfaces of the occipital lobes. Look into the space so produced between the cerebrum and cerebellum and, keeping close to the cerebellar surface, cut across the arachnoid and small vessels in the depths to reveal the tectum of the mid-brain with the colliculi (p. 38); the pineal body (p. 73) lies in the groove between the cranial pair of colliculi, and the slender fourth cranial nerves emerge just below the caudal pair. The end of the great cerebral vein (p. 111) can be identified immediately above the pineal body and below the splenium of the corpus callosum.

Remove carefully any remaining arachnoid mater over the interpeduncular fossa (p. 76) and so expose the cerebral peduncles (p. 39). Note their surface features and relationships, examine again the posterior cerebral, superior cerebellar and posteromedial and posterolateral central arteries (pp. 108, 109), and trace the basal vein (p. 110) as it winds round the midbrain to join the great cerebral vein or the commencement of the straight sinus. The third and fourth cranial nerves run forwards between the posterior cerebral and superior cerebellar arteries, the fourth immediately above the upper border of the pons. The optic tracts wind backwards to the geniculate bodies (p. 78) beneath the pulvinar of the thalamus (p. 69).

Next detach the brain-stem and cerebellum from the cerebrum as follows. Remove the vessels from the front and sides of the mid-brain, push the cerebrum and cerebellum apart by gentle pressure, and cut cleanly through the midbrain immediately above the colliculi and below the pineal body. In front the knife should emerge just below the interpeduncular (posterior) perforated substance to avoid damaging the corpora mamillaria. It is usually easier to section first one side and then the other, inserting the blade on the outer side and cutting towards the midline.

Strip off the larger vessels from the brain stem and cerebellum, preserving the third to the twelfth nerves if possible, although the delicate rootlets of the ninth to the twelfth nerves are often avulsed with the arachnoid.

The surface features of the medulla oblongata (pp. 31–33), pons (pp. 35–36), cerebellum (pp. 43–45) and midbrain (pp. 38–39) can now be examined. The middle cerebellar peduncles are easily seen, but the superior and inferior pair are best displayed by carefully separating the cerebellum and brain stem. The cranial medullary velum (p. 46) may be intact, but the caudal medullary velum (p. 46) is so thin that it usually tears during these manipulations. However it, or its remains, and the choroid plexus of the fourth ventricle should be identified. Normally there is an opening in the caudal velum, the median aperture of the roof of the fourth ventricle, or this part of the roof may be cribriform.

Now bisect the cerebellum in the median sagittal plane, avoiding damage to the floor of the fourth ventricle, and divide the three cerebellar peduncles on the left side so that this half of the cerebellum can be detached. This permits inspection of the cut surfaces of the cerebellum (p. 45) and of the fourth ventricle (pp. 46–48). If the floor of the ventricle cannot be seen properly the right cerebellar hemisphere should also be detached by cutting its peduncles. The structures described on pp. 47–48 can usually be easily recognised.

Make transverse sections through the midbrain, pons and medulla oblongata at about 1 cm intervals. The basis pedunculi, the substantia nigra, the red nucleus, the mesencephalic aqueduct and the mantle of grey matter around it, the transverse fibres of the pons with the intervening grey matter (pontine nuclei), the olivary nucleus and the central canal of the medulla can usually be identified; but other features such as the pyramidal and lemniscal fibres, the cranial nerve nuclei and so on are seldom easy to distinguish in unstained specimens. If available, therefore, sections of the brainstem stained by Weigert-Pal or other suitable techniques should be examined at this stage, preferably with the aid of a low-power lens.

The cerebrum

Remove any remaining arachnoid and pia mater from the surfaces of the hemispheres in order to facilitate examination of the sulci and gyri. Identify the surface features on the superolateral and inferior surfaces of the hemispheres (pp. 50, 55). The medial surface will be seen later. Separate the lips of the lateral fissure and examine the underlying insula (p. 52). Using a brain knife, cut off the top of the *right* cerebral hemisphere in a series of slices, each about 1 cm thick, down to the level of the upper part of the cingulate gyrus. Note the arrangement of the grey and white matter.

Remove the arachnoid and pia from the medial surface of the *left* hemisphere and study the sulci and gyri (pp. 53–55), and the anterior cerebral artery (p. 108). By blunt dissection try to expose the cingulum (p. 84), gradually scraping away the cortex and white matter above the genu of the corpus callosum and working backwards towards the splenium: the flattened bundle of fibres will be seen running from before backwards about 1 cm beneath the surface. The same scraping technique will reveal parts of the occipital (major) forceps and frontal (minor) forceps (p. 54). Blunt dissection is often facilitated by keeping the brain overnight in a refrigerator.

Running over the corpus callosum (p. 54) near the midline and just beneath the surface of the indusium griseum are the filiform medial and lateral longitudinal striae.

The lateral ventricles (pp. 80–82)

Make two transverse cuts 5 cm apart and 1 cm deep through the *right* cingulate gyrus and scoop out the intervening piece. The exposed surface consists of transverse callosal fibres and if it is palpated a lack of resistance will be noted, indicating the presence of a cavity beneath. Make a paramedial incision 2 cm from the midline through this thin region and separate the cut edges. The cavity revealed is the central part of the right lateral ventricle. Now remove the roof for about 1 cm on each side of the incision and identify the boundaries of this part of the ventricle. Having examined the central part of the ventricle, remove the roofs of the frontal and occipital horns by inserting a probe handle into each horn from the central part of the ventricle and cutting down on it. Take care when removing the roof of the occipital horn to avoid damage to the bulb of the occipital horn and the calcar avis.

Turn now to the medial surface of the *left* hemisphere and progressively scrape away the cortex and white matter over and above the cingulate gyrus. The ascending fibres of the corpus callosum will be seen rising into the hemisphere at an angle of about 45°; and the fibres of the cingulum can be traced as they pass backwards parallel to the corpus callosum before curving downwards behind the splenium. Slice off the top of the *left* cerebral hemisphere down to the upper surface of the corpus callosum. A slit will appear just to the left of the midline as the last cut is made. This is the left lateral ventricle and it should also be exposed and studied; the temporal horn will be examined later. Identify the septum pellucidum (p. 54), fornix (p. 67), bulb of posterior horn, calcar avis, choroidal fissure and choroid plexuses (p. 81). Note the caudate nucleus, thalamus, thalamostriate veins and stria terminalis in the floor of the central part of the ventricle.

Fornix and third ventricle (pp. 67–68 and 75–76)
Remove the trunk of the corpus callosum by cutting it at the genu and splenium and separating it carefully from the underlying fornix. The septum pellucidum, fornix and tela choroidea (p. 81) can now be seen more clearly. Insert the point of a scalpel through the interventricular foramina and cut upwards and forwards through the columns of the fornix. Reflect the fornix backwards, taking care not to displace the underlying tela choroidea, and divide the crura of the fornix; at this point the fornical commissure (p. 67–68) may be detected. The dissection should now show from before backwards: (1) the remains of the septum pellucidum, (2) the cut ends of the columns of the fornix forming the anterior boundaries of the interventricular foramina, (3) the interventricular foramina (p. 76), (4) the tela choroidea of the third ventricle (p. 76) with its edges forming the choroid plexuses of the lateral ventricles, and (5) the stria terminalis (p. 79) and thalamostriate veins in the groove between the caudate nucleus and thalamus.

Remove the remains of the splenium of the corpus callosum, and study the tela choroidea and the internal cerebral veins which unite posteriorly to form the great cerebral vein (p. 111). If the choroid plexuses are divided as they descend into the inferior horns of the lateral ventricles, the tela can be drawn upwards and forwards to expose the pineal body (p. 73) and the third ventricle (p. 75). The median double fringe attached to the under surface of the tela is the choroid plexus of the third ventricle. Note the posterior and habenular commissures (pp. 73 and 69), the stria medullaris thalami (stria habenularis) and the trigonum habenulae (p. 69). Turn the brain over to see the geniculate bodies (p. 73), the pulvinar (p. 69) and the optic tracts (p. 77). Replace the sections of the midbrain in their original positions and observe the rather indistinct brachia (p. 73) interconnecting the colliculi and the geniculate bodies.

Using a brain knife separate the two hemispheres by dividing all the remaining structures in the median sagittal plane. This is done by cutting straight downwards through the median slit of the third ventricle. It is now possible to identify many structures already described, such as: (1) the boundaries of the third ventricle, the thalamus, the stria medullaris thalami, the hypothalamic sulcus and parts of the hypothalamus, (2) parts of the corpus callosum, fornix and tela choroidea, (3) the optic chiasma, the tuber cinereum and infundibulum, the corpora mamillaria, the interpeduncular (posterior) perforated substance and the subthalamic tegmental region, (4) the lamina terminalis, the anterior commissure and the interventricular foramina, and (5) the pineal body and the posterior, habenular and fornical commissures. N.B. The hypophysis (pituitary gland) is seldom or never present in the brains available for dissection.

The rhinencephalon (pp. 66–69)
The olfactory bulb and tract, the rostral (anterior) perforated substance, the fornix, the indusium griseum, the longitudinal striae and the habenula have already been examined. Now identify the hippocampal sulcus, the parahippocampal gyrus and uncus and the narrow dentate gyrus (p. 67) which will be found lying deeply in the groove between the fimbria hippocampi and the parahippocampal gyrus. Separate the lips of the choroidal fissure (p. 81) and note the hippocampus (p. 67) and collateral eminence (p. 81) in the floor of the inferior horn of the lateral ventricle. To see these better the choroid plexus can be removed from the temporal horn.

Other features on the inferior surface of the cerebral hemisphere (pp. 55–56) should next be identified, such as the collateral and occipitotemporal sulci and the lingual and occipitotemporal gyri.

The thalamus and corpus striatum (pp. 69–73 and pp. 78–80)
Examine the thalamus again, and then in the remaining part of the left hemisphere make horizontal sections at 1 cm intervals, starting above, until the interthalamic adhesion is reached. Note the caudate and lentiform nuclei and the striated appearance created by the interconnections anteriorly; the division of the thalamus into three main parts by the internal medullary lamina; the internal capsule (p. 84); external capsule and claustrum (p. 79) and the insula (p. 52). The above sections open the frontal and occipital horns of the lateral

ventricle (p. 81); study the relationships of the caudate nucleus, corpus callosum and septum pellucidum to the former, and of the occipital (major) forceps and calcarine and collateral fissures to the latter.

Still using the *left* hemisphere, cut away the roof of the temporal horn of the lateral ventricle to expose more clearly the hippocampus and pes hippocampi (p. 67), the alveus, fimbria hippocampi and commencement of the crura of the fornix (p. 67), and the collateral eminence and trigone (p. 81). While removing the roof look carefully for the tail of the caudate nucleus, the amygdaloid body and the stria terminalis (p. 79).

Lastly make *coronal* sections through the remaining parts of the *right* hemisphere, starting at the frontal pole, and making each section about 2 cm thick. Study the cut surfaces as the sections pass backwards, identifying the insula, claustrum, external capsule, lentiform and caudate nuclei, internal capsule, optic tract, hippocampus, thalamus, and the various parts of the lateral ventricle and their boundaries.

SELECTED REFERENCES

The following works contain much more detailed information about the nervous system and should be consulted by those wishing to increase their knowledge.

Bourne, G. H. (Ed.) Vol. 1, 1968; Vol. II, 1969; Vol. III, 1969; Vol. IV, 1972; Vol. V, 1972; Vol. VI, 1972. *Structure and Function of Nervous Tissue.* New York: Academic Press.

Brodal, A. (1957) *The Reticular Formation of the Brain Stem.* Edinburgh: Oliver & Boyd.

Brodal, A. (1981) *Neurological Anatomy in Relation to Clinical Medicine.* 3rd Ed. New York: Oxford University Press.

Bülbring, E. (Ed.) (1970) Smooth Muscle. London: Arnold.

Burnstock, G. & Costa, M. (1975) *Adrenergic Neurones, their Organisation, Function, and Development in the Peripheral Nervous System.* London: Chapman & Hall.

Crosby, E. D., Humphrey, T. & Lauer, E. W. (1962) *Correlative Anatomy of the Nervous System.* New York: Macmillan.

Curtis, B. A, Jacobson, S. &Marcus, E. M. (1972) *An Introduction to the Neurosciences.* Philadelphia: Saunders.

Eccles, J. C. (1964) *The Physiology of Synapses.* Berlin: Springer.

Eccles, J. C. (1972) *The Understanding of the Brain.* New York: McGraw-Hill.

Eccles, J. C., Ito, M. & Szentagothai, J. (1967) *The Cerebellum as a Neurone Machine.* Berlin: Springer.

Kandel, E. R. & Schwartz, J. H. (1981) *Principles of Neural Science.* New York, Elsevier North-Holland.

Kapper, C. U. A., Huber, G. C. & Crosby, E. C. (1936) *The Comparative Anatomy of the Nervous System of Vertebrates, including Man.* New York: Macmillan.

Magoun, H. W. (1958) *The Waking Brain*. Springfield, Illinois: Thomas.

Miller, R. A. & Burack, E. (1968) *Atlas of the Central Nervous System in Man*. Baltimore: Williams & Wilkins.

Mitchell, G. A. G. (1953) *Anatomy of the Autonomic Nervous System*. Edinburgh: Livingstone.

Mitchell, G. A. G. (1956) *Cardiovascular Innervation*. Edinburgh: Livingstone.

Netter, F. H. (1953) *The Nervous System*. Ciba Collection of Medical Illustrations, Vol. 1.

Penfield, W. & Rasmussen, T. (1950) *The Cerebral Cortex of Man*. New York: Macmillan.

Pick, J. (1970) *The Autonomic Nervous System*. Philadelphia: Lippincott.

Ranson, S. W. & Clark, S. L. (1959) *The Anatomy of the Nervous System*. Philadelphia: Saunders.

Refsum, S. *et al*. (Eds.) (1963) The so-called extrapyramidal system. *Acta Neurologia Scandinavica*, **Vol. 39**, Suppl. 4.

Russell, W. R. (1959) *Brain, Memory, Learning*. Oxford: Clarendon Press.

Schmitt, F. O. (Ed.) (1967) *The Neurosciences: A Study Program*. New York: Rockefeller U. P.

Schmitt, F. O. (Ed.) (1971) *The Neurosciences: Second Study Program*. New York: Rockefeller U. P.

Schmitt, F. O. & Worden, F. G. (Eds.) (1974) *The Neurosciences: Third Study Program*. Cambridge, Mass: MIT Press.

Schmitt, F. O. & Worden, F. G. (Eds) (1979) *The neurosciences: Fourth Study Program*. Cambridge, Mass: MIT Press.

Sherrington, C. S. (1947) *The Integrative Action of the Nervous System*. London: Cambridge University Press.

Smythies, J. R. (Ed.) (1965) *Brain and Mind*. London: Routledge & Kegan Paul.

Truex, R. C. & Carpenter, M. B. (1969) *Human Neuroanatomy*. Baltimore: Williams & Wilkins.

Walshe, F. M. R. (1948) *Critical Studies in Neurology*. Edinburgh: Livingstone.

Index